改訂版 クインテッセンス歯科英会話シリーズ

英語で話す歯科受付！

PART 3

ENGLISH CONVERSATION FOR RECEPTIONIST-PATIENT COMMUNICATION

Thomas R. Ward 著

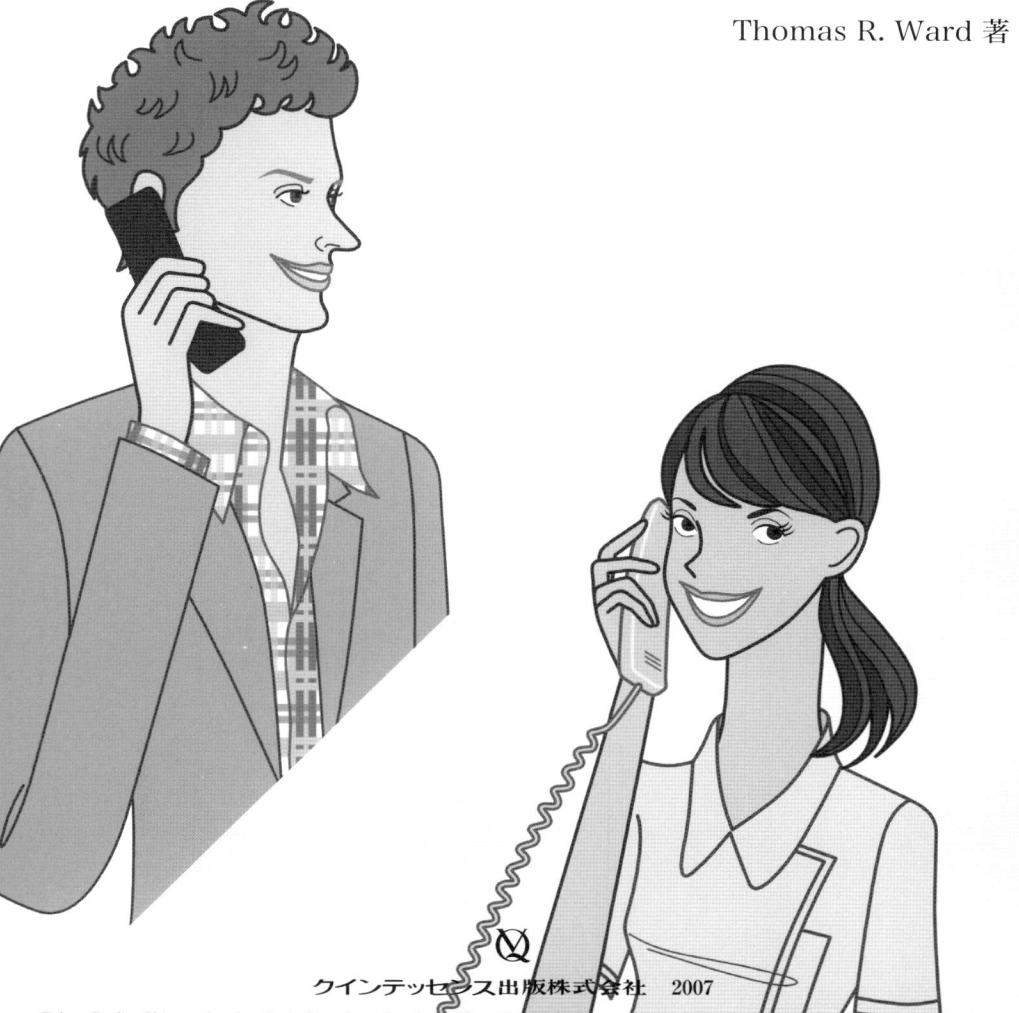

クインテッセンス出版株式会社　2007

Tokyo, Berlin, Chicago, London, Paris, Barcelona, Istanbul, Milano, São Paulo, Moscow, Prague, Warsaw, New Delhi, Beijing, and Bukarest

まえがき

　本書は、歯科医院の受付係やスタッフが外国人患者とのコミュニケーションを持つ際に手助けになるように書かれたもである。現在、日本には200万人以上の外国人が在住しているが、それに加え、毎年700万人を越える人々が日本を訪れている。日本の国際化の証拠となるものだが、この数はますます増えていくようである。この外国人たちは、教師、ビジネスマン、外交官、開発途上国からの留学生など、さまざまな職業や国籍の人々である。

　受付係やスタッフとこうした外国人患者とのコミュニケーションを図るうえで、いろいろな問題が起こりかねない。一般的に言って外国人は、日本人に比べて自分の受ける治療の説明を求めることが多いようである。また、国や職業の違いのため、患者が歯科治療に何を期待しているか、はっきりとつかみにくいこともある。本書では、受付係やスタッフが日常の診療で、外国人患者と話すときに役立つような、基本的会話を集めてみた。

　なお、本書の出版に際しては、クインテッセンス出版の佐々木一高氏にアドバイス、ご教示をいただいた。ここに書面をかりて御礼申し上げる次第である。

Thomas R. Ward

本書の使用にあたって

　本書は、独学にも、また教室での勉強にも使用できる。歯科診療所で外国人患者と接する際の日常的なシチュエーションで、アポイント、支払いなどを説明する基本的な対話を集めた。本書は10章からなり、それぞれ2つのセクションに分かれている。最初は患者との対話で、一般の人にもわかる平易な用語で歯科の1つのトピックを説明している。この対話では専門用語は使っていない。各章の対話の前には、場面の説明を簡単にしているが、この中には、歯科医やスタッフだけが使う専門用語が含まれていることもある。

　第2のセクションは、対話中の文章を使った5つの入れ換え練習問題がある。ここに使われている用語には、専門的な性格のもの（歯周病など）、患者が理解できる言葉（むし歯、クラウンなど）もある。この問題は、マスターするまで反復練習をするとよいだろう。

　本書の最後には、受付係やスタッフと患者とのコミュニケーションのための、もっとも重要な100語を載せた。これらはすべて歯科用語を特に知らない人にでもわかる言葉である。このような言葉は、患者とのコミュニケーションに欠かせないものなので、対話の勉強を始める前に暗記するのも良いだろう。

　なお、本書を活かすためには、収録した音声を併用して学習することを勧める。

CD（収録音声）の使い方

　本書とセットになったCDには、次のものが収録されている。①各章の英会話すべて、②各章の練習問題の例題すべて、③各章の練習問題の置き換え語句の一部（特に発音が難しいと思われるもの）。

１．各章の英会話を練習する順序と方法
①まず、会話全体をとおして聞いてみる。
②発音と意味がわかったところで、実際に声を出して会話を模倣する。この際、１人が話す度ごとに音声を止め、反復練習をしてみると効果的である。
③次に、自分が対話の一方の役になって、その部分を言ってみる。たとえば、登場している歯科受付になったつもりで、患者の発音ごとに音声を止め、歯科受付の応答文を言ってみる。次いで音声を再開し、自分の発音、イントネーションが正しいかどうか確認する。この役割練習は、歯科受付だけでなく、患者にもなって行うべきである。
④次に双方の役割を１人でこなして、全文を暗記してみる。この際、会話にあるイントネーションを意識的にまねてみることが重要である。

２．練習問題の使い方
①例題と語句の置き換わったものを２～３回聞き、声を出して反復練習してみる。
②発音とイントネーションを耳と口が覚えたと思ったら、練習問題の置き換え語句を入れ換えて、次々声を出して練習してみる。
③その際、１つずつ置き換え語句ごとに音声を止め、声を出して置き換えられた文を発音してみる。
④置き換え文章を12まで発音し終わったら、また１まで戻り、置き換えがスムーズに言えるようにする。
⑤置き換えがスムーズに言えるようになったら、自分で置き換え語句を考え出し、どんどん置き換え文を作ってみる。自分の毎日の仕事と職場を想定し、いろいろ楽しい置き換え文を作ってみよう。

　以上、短時間でも繰り返し行ってみよう。英会話の習得は、納得のいくまで声を出して練習することがコツである。

CONTENTS

まえがき ……………………………………………………… 3

本書の使用にあたって ……………………………… 4

CD（収録音声）の使い方 ……………………………… 5

第1章　電話の応対 Ⅰ．新患のためのアポイント …… 8 　　I Would Like to Make an Appointment. 　　予約をしたいのですが

第2章　電話の応対 Ⅱ．救急のアポイント …………… 20 　　The Tooth Is Killing Me. 　　歯が痛くて死にそうです

第3章　電話の応対 Ⅲ．道を教える ……………………… 32 　　Can You Give Me Directions to the Office? 　　診療所へ行く道を教えてくださいますか？

第4章　電話の応対 Ⅳ．診療費に関する質問 ………… 46 　　How Much Will It Cost? 　　おいくらぐらいかかりますか？

第5章　電話の応対 Ⅴ．アポイントのキャンセル ……… 58
　　I Am Too Busy to Keep My Appointment This Afternoon.
　　とても忙しくて、午後の予約時間に行けないんですが

第6章　電話の応対 Ⅵ．医師への電話 …………………… 70
　　May I Talk with the Doctor?
　　先生とお話できますか？

第7章　患者へのあいさつ ………………………………… 82
　　I Am Afraid It Has Been a Long Time Since My Last Checkup.
　　この前の検診からずいぶんたったようですね

第8章　外国の保険の用紙に書き入れる ………………… 94
　　Does The Dentist Accept This Insurance?
　　先生はこの保険を受けていらっしゃいますか？

第9章　請求業務 …………………………………………… 106
　　Could You Send the Bill to My Office?
　　請求書は私の事務所の方に送っていただけますか

第10章　治療記録を患者に渡す …………………………… 118
　　Could I Have a Copy of My Dental Records?
　　私の歯科記録のコピーをいただけますか？

付録 ………………………………………………………… 132
　　患者とのコミュニケーションで役立つ最重要用語100語

Chapter 1

Use of the telephone
Part I : An appointment for a new patient

I Would Like to Make an Appointment.

The initial telephone conversation is very important since this is the first contact most patients will have with your office. It is important to be polite and speak clearly. Do not forget to ask for the patient's telephone number in case future contact is necessary.

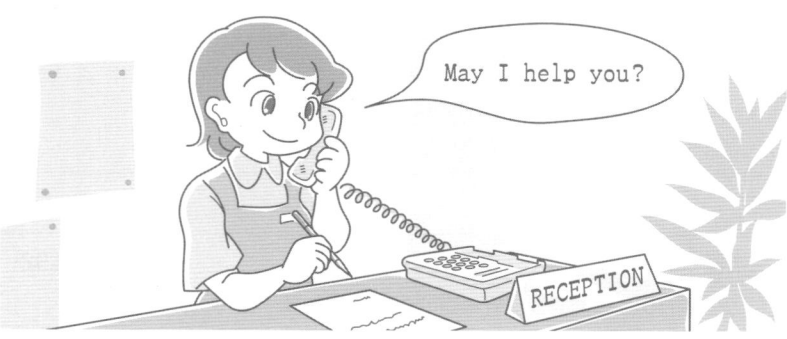

第 1 章

電話の応対
Ⅰ. 新患のためのアポイント

予約をしたいのですが

　ほとんどの患者は最初に電話で診療所に連絡してくるので、最初の電話応対は非常に大切である。礼儀正しく、はっきりと話すことが大切である。後で連絡する必要がある時に備えて、患者の電話番号を尋ねるのを忘れてはいけない。

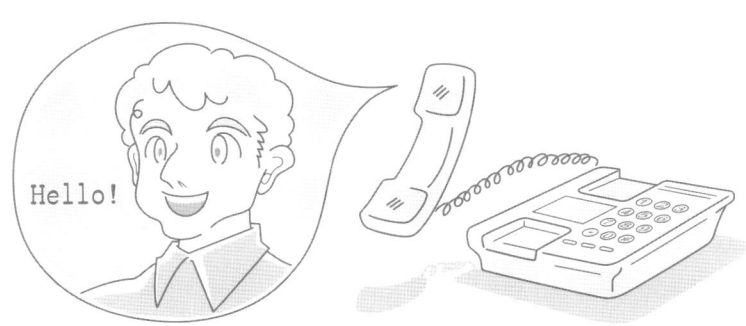

Situation: Mr. Ferme, an Italian merchant is calling the clinic to make an appointment for a checkup and cleaning.

Ms. Fukuoka: Good morning. This is the Hayashi Dental Clinic. May I help you?
Mr. Ferme: I would like to make an appointment for a checkup and cleaning.
Ms. Fukuoka: Certainly, when would be convenient for you?
Mr. Ferme: Would tomorrow morning be acceptable?
Ms. Fukuoka: I am sorry but the doctor is busy all morning. Could you come in Friday morning?

Mr. Ferme: That would be fine. What time is available?
Ms. Fukuoka: Either nine or eleven.
Mr. Ferme: In that case, would you put me down for nine o'clock?
Ms. Fukuoka: Certainly. May I have your name and telephone number?
Mr. Ferme: The name is Ferme.
Ms. Fukuoka: Could you spell it please?
Mr. Ferme: Ferme, F − E − R − M − E.
Ms. Fukuoka: And the telephone number, please?
Mr. Ferme: One, seven, nine, six, nine, eight, nine.
Ms. Fukuoka: Thank you. We will be expecting you Friday morning at nine o'clock.
Mr. Ferme: Thank you. Good bye.
Ms. Fukuoka: Good bye.

場面：イタリア人商人のフェルメ氏が、検診とクリーニングのアポイントを取るために診療所に電話をかけている。

福岡さん：おはようございます。林歯科医院でございます。

フェルメ氏：検診とクリーニングの予約をしたいのですが。

福岡さん：かしこまりました。いつがご都合よろしいでしょうか。
フェルメ氏：明日の午前中はよいでしょうか。
福岡さん：申し訳ございませんが、先生は午前中ずっとつまっております。金曜日の午前中に来ていただけますでしょうか。
フェルメ氏：それで結構です。何時があいていますか？
福岡さん：9時か11時です。
フェルメ氏：それなら、9時に取っておいてください。

福岡さん：かしこまりました。お名前とお電話番号をいただけますか。
フェルメ氏：名前はフェルメです。
福岡さん：つづりを言っていただけますか。
フェルメ氏：フェルメ、F-E-R-M-E。
福岡さん：お電話番号をお願いします。
フェルメ氏：179-6989
福岡さん：ありがとうございます。金曜日の午前9時にお待ちしております。
フェルメ氏：ありがとう。さようなら。
福岡さん：失礼いたします。

Exercises

Ⅰ. Substitute the following expressions in the example sentence.

It is important to <u>be polite</u>.
⟨see the dentist every six months⟩
It is important to <u>see the dentist every six months</u>.

1. have your teeth cleaned
2. be on time for the appointment
3. brush every day
4. use floss every day
5. brush and floss daily
6. have regular checkups
7. remove the plaque
8. remove all the stain from the teeth
9. remove the calculus from the teeth
10. have X-rays every six months
11. visit the dentist regularly
12. find a good dentist

Ⅱ. Substitute the following expressions in the example sentence.

Do not forget to ask for the patient's <u>phone number</u>.
⟨chief complaint⟩
Do not forget to ask for the patient's <u>chief complaint</u>.

練習問題

Ⅰ．例文の下線部を以下の語句に置き換えなさい。

<u>礼儀正しくする</u>ことは大切である。
〈6ヵ月ごとに歯医者に行く〉
<u>6ヵ月ごとに歯医者に行く</u>ことは大切である。

1. 歯をクリーニングしてもらう
2. アポイントの時間を守る
3. 毎日磨く
4. 毎日フロスを使う
5. 毎日磨いてフロスする
6. 定期検診を受ける
7. プラークを取り除く
8. その歯からステインを取り除く
9. その歯から歯石を取り除く
10. 6ヵ月ごとにエックス線写真を撮る
11. 定期的に歯医者を訪れる
12. よい歯医者をみつける

Ⅱ．例文の下線部を以下の語句に置き換えなさい。

患者の<u>電話番号</u>を尋ねるのを忘れないように。
〈主訴〉
患者の<u>主訴</u>を尋ねるのを忘れないように。

1. home address
2. office address
3. home telephone number
4. office telephone number
5. physical condition
6. health history
7. history of present illness
8. family health history
9. reason for seeking treatment
10. reason for wanting dentures
11. reason for coming to the clinic
12. reason for desiring a crown

Ⅲ. Substitute the following expressions in the example sentence.

He would like to make an appointment for a checkup.
⟨to see the hygienist⟩
He would like to make an appointment to see the hygienist.

1. for an examination
2. for removal of calculus
3. to have the calculus removed
4. to have his teeth examined
5. for his annual checkup
6. for brushing instructions
7. to consult with the hygienist
8. to continue treatment

1. 自宅の住所
2. 勤務先の住所
3. 自宅の電話番号
4. 勤務先の電話番号
5. 身体の状態
6. 既往歴
7. 現在かかっている病気の経過
8. 家族の既往歴
9. 治療を求める理由
10. 義歯がほしい理由
11. 診療所に来る理由
12. クラウンがほしい理由

Ⅲ．例文の下線部を以下の語句に置き換えなさい。

彼は検診のためにアポイントを取りたい。
〈歯科衛生士に診てもらうために〉
彼は歯科衛生士に診てもらうためにアポイントを取りたい。

1. 診察のために
2. 歯石除去のために
3. 歯石を除去してもらうために
4. 歯を診察してもらうために
5. １年ごとの定期検診のために
6. ブラッシング指導のために
7. 歯科衛生士と相談するために
8. 治療を続けるために

9. to get a crown
10. to have the filling replaced
11. for a crown
12. for a filling

Ⅳ. Substitute the following expressions in the example dialogue.

- When would you like to <u>come here</u>?
- Any time would be OK.

⟨visit here⟩

- When would you like to <u>visit here</u>?
- Any time would be OK.

1. come to the office
2. get instructions on brushing and flossing
3. have the tooth filled
4. reschedule the appointment
5. have your teeth cleaned
6. visit your dentist
7. make an appointment
8. see the dentist
9. see the hygienist
10. make an appointment with the dentist
11. make an appointment with the hygienist
12. come to the clinic

9. クラウンをしてもらうために
10. 充填物を取りかえてもらうために
11. クラウンのために
12. 充填のために

Ⅳ．例にあげた対話の下線部を以下の語句に置き換えなさい。

－いつ、ここにおいでになりたいですか。
－いつでも結構です。
〈ここを訪ねる〉
－いつ、ここをお訪ねになりたいですか。
－いつでも結構です。

1. 診療所に来る
2. ブラッシングとフロッシング指導を受ける
3. 歯を充填してもらう
4. 予約を変更する
5. 歯をクリーニングしてもらう
6. 歯医者を訪ねる
7. 予約をする
8. 歯医者に診てもらう
9. 歯科衛生士に診てもらう
10. 歯医者の予約をする
11. 歯科衛生士の予約をする
12. 診療所に来る

Ⅴ. Substitute the following expressions in the example dialogue.

- May I have your name?
- The name is <u>Ferme</u>.
- Could you spell it please?
- <u>Ferme, F - E - R - M - E</u>.

⟨Ward⟩
- May I have your name?
- The name is <u>Ward</u>.
- Could you spell it please?
- <u>Ward, W - A - R - D</u>.

1. Sawada
2. Smith
3. Jones
4. Johnson
5. Slocum
6. Given
7. Booth
8. Patten
9. Boyd
10. Heart
11. Bush
12. Reagan

Ⅴ．例にあげた対話の下線部を以下の語句に置き換えなさい。

－お名前をいただけますか。
－名前は<u>フェルメ</u>です。
－つづりを言っていただけますか。
－<u>フェルメ、F－E－R－M－E</u>。
〈ウォード〉
－お名前をいただけますか。
－名前は<u>ウォード</u>です。
－つづりを言っていただけますか。
－<u>ウォード、W－A－R－D</u>。

1. サワダ
2. スミス
3. ジョーンズ
4. ジョンソン
5. スローカム
6. ギブン
7. ブース
8. パッテン
9. ボイド
10. ハート
11. ブッシュ
12. レーガン

Chapter 2

Use of the telephone
Part II: An appointment for an emergency

The Tooth Is Killing Me.

The most important thing with an emergency patient is to determine if the condition is really an emergency or not. If the patient has a chipped tooth which has been chipped for two months and he is not in pain, he can be scheduled any time. However, if the patient is in pain, it is important to see him as soon as possible.

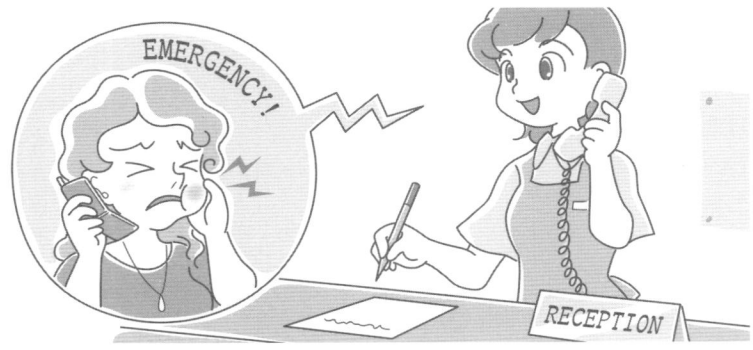

第 2 章

電話の応対
Ⅱ. 救急のアポイント

歯が痛くて死にそうです

　急患でもっとも大切なのは、その状態が本当に緊急なものかどうか見極めることである。もし、2ヵ月も前に欠けた歯で、しかも痛くないのであれば、いつアポイントを入れてもよい。しかし、もし痛みがあれば、できるだけすぐにその患者を診ることが大切である。

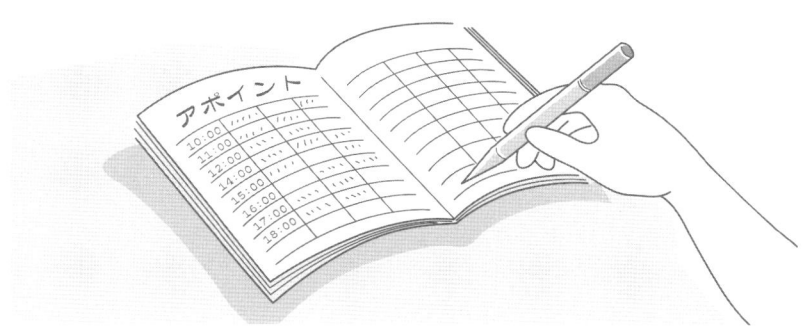

Situation: Lisa Miller, a Canadian English teacher, is calling for an appointment. She has a bad toothache and needs immediate treatment.

Ms. Fukuoka: Good morning. This is the Hayashi Dental Clinic. May I help you?
Ms. Miller: I would like an appointment as soon as possible.
Ms. Fukuoka: Would next Monday at three o'clock be acceptable?
Ms. Miller: Actually, I have a bad toothache. Could the doctor see me sooner?
Ms. Fukuoka: He is quite busy today but he may be able to see you briefly at two o'clock.
Ms. Miller: That would be fine.
Ms. Fukuoka: Could I have your name and phone number, please?
Ms. Miller: Miller, M−I−L−L−E−R.
Ms. Fukuoka: Thank you. And the phone number, please.
Ms. Miller: One, two, three, eight, seven, six, eight.
Ms. Fukuoka: Thank you.
Ms. Miller: Will the doctor be able to finish the treatment today?
Ms. Fukuoka: He is very busy today and may not be able to finish all of the treatment. But at least he should be able to relieve the pain.
Ms. Miller: I hope so. The tooth is killing me. I will be at the office at two.
Ms. Fukuoka: Thank you for calling. Good bye.
Ms. Miller: Good bye.

場面：カナダ人の英語の教師、リサ・ミラーはアポイントのために電話をかけている。ひどい歯痛があり、すぐに治療する必要がある。

 福岡さん：おはようございます。林歯科医院でございます。

ミラーさん：できるだけすぐに予約をしたいのですが。
 福岡さん：来週の月曜日、3時でよろしいでしょうか。
ミラーさん：実は、ひどい歯痛なんです。もっと早く先生に診ていただけませんか。
 福岡さん：先生は、今日とても忙しいのですが、少しの間でしたら2時に診ることができるかもしれません。
ミラーさん：それで結構です。
 福岡さん：お名前とお電話番号をいただけますか。

ミラーさん：ミラー、M－I－L－L－E－R。
 福岡さん：ありがとうございます。お電話番号をお願いします。
ミラーさん：123－8768
 福岡さん：ありがとうございます。
ミラーさん：先生は、今日治療を終えることができますか。

 福岡さん：今日は、大変忙しいので、治療を全部終えることはできないかもしれません。でも、少なくとも痛みをやわらげることはできるはずです。
ミラーさん：そうだといいですわ。歯が痛くて死にそうなんです。診療所に2時に参ります。
 福岡さん：お電話ありがとうございました。失礼いたします。
ミラーさん：さようなら。

Exercises

Ⅰ. Substitute the following expressions in the example sentence.

Determine if the condition is <u>really an emergency</u>.
⟨really bad⟩
Determine if the condition is <u>really bad</u>.

1. serious
2. important
3. painful
4. very painful
5. very serious
6. going to require an appointment immediately
7. hopeless
8. beyond repair
9. beyond hope
10. dangerous
11. dangerous for the patient's health
12. of any importance

Ⅱ. Substitute the following expressions in the example sentence.

The patient needs <u>immediate treatment</u>.
⟨to see the dentist⟩
The patient needs <u>to see the dentist</u>.

練習問題

Ⅰ．例文の下線部を以下の語句に置き換えなさい。

その状態が本当に緊急なものであるかどうか見極めなさい。
〈本当に悪い〉
その状態が本当に悪いかどうか見極めなさい。

1. 重大である
2. 大切である
3. 痛い
4. 非常に痛い
5. 非常に重大である
6. アポイントをすぐに取る必要がある
7. 見込みがない
8. 修理ができない
9. 望みがない
10. 危険である
11. 患者の健康にとって危険である
12. 少しでも重要である

Ⅱ．例文の下線部を以下の語句に置き換えなさい。

その患者はすぐに治療することが必要だ。
〈歯医者に診てもらう〉
その患者は歯医者に診てもらう必要がある。

1. a new denture
2. a crown
3. to get a new filling
4. to have a consultation
5. to receive brushing instructions
6. a thorough cleaning
7. additional treatment
8. a plastic filling
9. a partial denture
10. to see a specialist
11. to have his X-rays
12. an appointment

Ⅲ. Substitute the following expressions in the example sentence.

Will the doctor be able to <u>finish the treatment</u> today?
⟨see me⟩
Will the doctor be able to <u>see me</u> today?

1. finish the work
2. do the crown
3. talk with me
4. keep the appointment
5. start the treatment
6. do the root canal treatment
7. complete the treatment
8. finish the root canal treatment

1. 新しい義歯
2. クラウン
3. 新しい充填をしてもらう
4. 相談をする
5. 歯ブラシ指導を受ける
6. 徹底的なクリーニング
7. 付加的な治療
8. プラスチックの充填
9. 部分義歯
10. 専門医に診てもらう
11. エックス線写真を撮る
12. アポイント

Ⅲ．例文の下線部を以下の語句に置き換えなさい。

先生は、今日治療を終えることができますか。
〈私を診る〉
先生は、今日私を診ることができますか。

1. その仕事を終える
2. クラウンをする
3. 私と話す
4. アポイントを守る
5. 治療を始める
6. 根管治療をする
7. 治療を終える
8. 根管治療を終える

9. talk with the hygienist
10. clean my teeth
11. take the X-ray
12. give me my X-rays

Ⅳ. Substitute the following expressions in the example sentence.

The doctor may be able to <u>see you</u> later.
⟨do the treatment⟩
The doctor may be able to <u>do the treatment</u> later.

1. talk with you
2. come to the phone
3. begin the treatment
4. have the treatment plan ready
5. do the work
6. start work on the crown
7. treat the patient
8. consult with the patient
9. return your phone call
10. see the emergency patient
11. talk with the hygienist
12. find the cause of your pain

9. 歯科衛生士と話す
10. 私の歯をクリーニングする
11. エックス線写真を撮る
12. 私のエックス線写真をくださる

Ⅳ．例文の下線部を以下の語句に置き換えなさい。

先生は、後ほどあなたを診ることができるかもしれません。
〈治療をする〉
先生は、後ほど治療をすることができるかもしれません。

1. あなたと話す
2. 電話に出る
3. 治療を始める
4. 治療計画を準備する
5. 仕事をする
6. クラウンの仕事を始める
7. 患者を治療する
8. 患者と相談する
9. あなたに電話をかけ直す
10. 急患を診る
11. 歯科衛生士と話す
12. 痛みの原因をみつける

Ⅴ. Substitute the following expressions in the example sentence.

Actually I have a bad toothache.
⟨a bad headache⟩
Actually I have a bad headache.

1. periodontal problems
2. sore spots under the denture
3. gum disease
4. loose dentures
5. a loose crown
6. a broken filling
7. bleeding gums
8. a broken tooth
9. a loose tooth
10. a sharp pain in one of my teeth
11. sore gums
12. a loose partial denture

Ⅴ．例文の下線部を以下の語句に置き換えなさい。

実は、ひどい歯痛があるのです。
〈ひどい頭痛〉
実は、ひどい頭痛があるのです。

 1. 歯周病の問題
 2. 義歯の下に痛む箇所
 3. 歯ぐきの病気
 4. 義歯に緩み
 5. クラウンに緩み
 6. 割れた充填物
 7. 歯ぐきから出血
 8. 割れた歯
 9. ぐらぐらする歯
10. 歯に鋭い痛み
11. 歯ぐきの痛み
12. 部分義歯に緩み

Chapter 3

Use of the telephone
Part Ⅲ: Giving directions

Can You Give Me Directions to the Office?

When giving directions, speak clearly and repeat yourself often. It is a good idea to write out the directions in English and place them near the telephone so that you can read them to the person who is calling. Tell the patient to bring along your office phone number in case he gets lost on the way to the office.

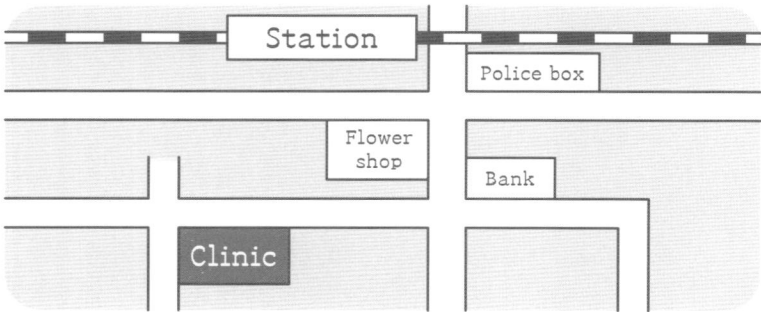

第3章

電話の応対
Ⅲ．道を教える

診療所へ行く道を教えてくださいますか？

　道を教える時は、はっきりと話し何度も繰り返すこと。英語で道順を書き電話の近くにおいて、電話をかけてくる人にそれを読んであげられるようにしておくのもよい。もし患者が診療所に来る途中で迷った時のために、診療所の電話番号を持ってくるように言ってあげる。

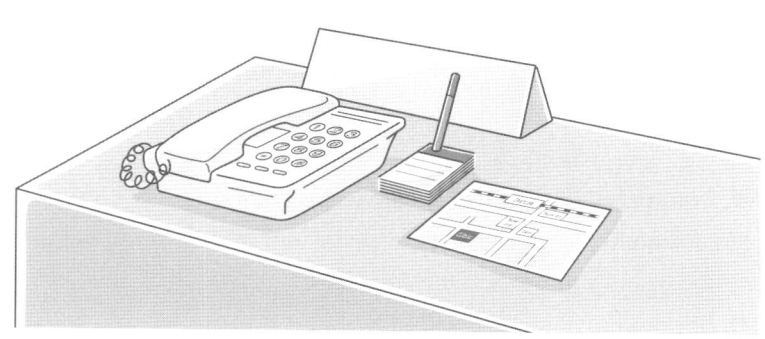

Situation: Mr. Johanson who called earlier for an appointment, is calling back to get directions to the office.

Ms. Fukuoka: Good evening. This is the Hayashi Dental Clinic. May I help you?
Mr. Johanson: This is Johanson. I called this morning for an appointment.
Ms. Fukuoka: Hello Mr. Johanson. What can I do for you?
Mr. Johanson: Can you give me directions to the office?
Ms. Fukuoka: Certainly. Do you know how to get to Meguro Station?
Mr. Johanson: Yes. It is on the Yamanote line, isn't it?
Ms. Fukuoka: Yes. From Meguro Station go out the west exit.
Mr. Johanson: OK.
Ms. Fukuoka: In front of the exit is a large department store. Turn right as you leave the exit and go north two blocks.
Mr. Johanson: Is there a landmark at that corner?
Ms. Fukuoka: Yes, there is a police box on the corner. Turn left at this corner.
Mr. Johanson: OK.
Ms. Fukuoka: Go down this street one hundred meters. On the left hand side is a large sign which says, "The Hayashi Dental Clinic."
Mr. Johanson: Thank you. I should be able to find it.
Ms. Fukuoka: You might take along our phone number in case there is some problem.
Mr. Johanson: That is a good idea.

場面：ジョハンソン氏は前にアポイントのために電話したのだが、診療所への道を尋ねるためにもう一度電話をしている。

　　　福岡さん：こんばんは。林歯科医院でございます。

ジョハンソン：こちらはジョハンソンです。今朝、予約を取るために電話した者ですが。
　　　福岡さん：ジョハンソンさん、どういったご用件でしょうか。
ジョハンソン：診療所に行く道を教えてくださいますか。
　　　福岡さん：かしこまりました。目黒駅への行き方はご存知ですか。
ジョハンソン：ええ。山の手線ですね。
　　　福岡さん：はい。目黒駅から、西口に出てください。
ジョハンソン：OK．
　　　福岡さん：出口の正面に大きいデパートがあります。出口を出て右に曲がり、北に2ブロック行ってください。

ジョハンソン：その角には目印がありますか？
　　　福岡さん：はい。角には交番があります。そこを左に曲がってください。
ジョハンソン：OK．
　　　福岡さん：その道を100メートル行ってください。左側に大きな看板があって、林歯科医院と書いてあります。

ジョハンソン：ありがとう。それでみつけられると思います。
　　　福岡さん：もし何か問題があった時のために、私どもの電話番号をお持ちになるといいかもしれません。
ジョハンソン：それはよい考えですね。

Ms. Fukuoka: We are looking forward to seeing you next Wednesday at ten o'clock.
Mr. Johanson: Thank you. Good bye.
Ms. Fukuoka: Good bye.

福岡さん：来週水曜日の10時においでになるのをお待ちしております。
ジョハンソン：ありがとう。さようなら。
福岡さん：失礼いたします。

Exercises

I. Substitute the following expressions in the example sentence.

Mr. Johanson is calling to <u>get directions to the office</u>.
⟨talk with the dentist⟩
Mr. Johanson is calling to <u>talk with the dentist</u>.

1. make an appointment
2. talk with the hygienist
3. talk with the office manager
4. ask about fees
5. check his appointment time
6. confirm his appointment
7. schedule an appointment
8. reschedule his appointment
9. cancel his appointment
10. get some information
11. see if he can get an appointment
12. see if the doctor is free to talk on the phone

II. Substitute the following expressions in the example dialogue.

— Can you give me directions to <u>the office</u>?
— Certainly. I'll be glad to.
⟨the dentist's office⟩
— Can you give me directions to <u>the dentist's office</u>?

練習問題

I．例文の下線部を以下の語句に置き換えなさい。

ジョハンソン氏は診療所への道を尋ねるために電話している。
〈歯医者と話す〉
ジョハンソン氏は歯医者と話すために電話している。

1. アポイントを取る
2. 歯科衛生士と話す
3. オフィスのマネージャーと話す
4. 診療費について尋ねる
5. アポイントの時間をチェックする
6. アポイントを確認する
7. アポイントを入れる
8. アポイントを変更する
9. アポイントをキャンセルする
10. 何かを聞くために
11. アポイントが取れるかどうか聞く
12. 先生が電話で話せるかどうか聞く

II．例にあげた対話の下線部を以下の語句に置き換えなさい。

－診療所に行く道を教えてくださいますか。
－はい。喜んで。
〈歯科医院〉
－歯科医院に行く道を教えてくださいますか。

−Certainly. I'll be glad to.

1. the police box closest to your office
2. the orthodontist's office
3. the doctor's office
4. the specialist's office
5. the office from my home
6. her office
7. your office
8. your dental clinic
9. the nearest station to your office
10. the drugstore by your office
11. the pharmacy closest to your office
12. give the taxi driver

Ⅲ. Substitute the following expressions in the example dialogue.

−Do you know how to get to <u>Meguro Station</u>?
−I think I can find it.
⟨this office⟩
−Do you know how to get to <u>this office</u>?
−I think I can find it.

1. IBM headquarters
2. Roppongi
3. the dentist's clinic
4. the specialist's office

－はい。喜んで。

1. 診療所に一番近い交番
2. 矯正医の診療所
3. 先生の診療所
4. 専門医の診療所
5. 私の家から診療所
6. 彼女の診療所
7. あなたの診療所
8. あなたの歯科診療所
9. あなたの診療所に一番近い駅
10. 診療所の近くの薬局
11. 診療所に一番近い薬局
12. タクシーの運転手に教えるため

Ⅲ．例にあげた対話の下線部を以下の語句に置き換えなさい。

－目黒駅への行き方はご存知ですか。
－わかると思います。
〈こちらの診療所〉
－こちらの診療所への行き方はご存知ですか。
－わかると思います。

1. IBM本部
2. 六本木
3. 歯科診療所
4. 専門医の診療所

5. my office

6. the doctor's office

7. this building

8. the subway stop nearest this office

9. Shinjuku Station

10. the police box nearest our office

11. the main intersection by our office

12. the train station by our office

Ⅳ. Substitute the following expressions in the example sentence.

We are looking forward to seeing you.
〈your call〉
We are looking forward to your call.

1. your appointment

2. beginning your treatment

3. visiting your office

4. meeting your family

5. hearing from you

6. receiving your phone call

7. seeing your children

8. continuing the treatment

9. completing the treatment

10. hearing from Dr. Yamamoto

11. meeting you

12. your next visit

5. 私の診療所
6. 先生の診療所
7. このビル
8. 診療所から一番近い地下鉄の駅
9. 新宿駅
10. 診療所から一番近い交番
11. 診療所の近くの大きな交差点
12. 診療所から近い駅

Ⅳ．例文の下線部を以下の語句に置き換えなさい。

<u>あなたにお会いする</u>のを楽しみにしています。
〈あなたのお電話〉
<u>あなたのお電話</u>をお待ちしています。

1. あなたの予約
2. あなたの治療を始める
3. あなたの診療所を訪れる
4. あなたのご家族にお会いする
5. あなたからのお便り
6. あなたからのお電話
7. あなたのお子さんたちにお会いする
8. 治療を続ける
9. 治療を終える
10. 山本先生からお便りをいただく
11. あなたにお会いする
12. あなたが次に来られる

V. Substitute the following expressions in the example sentence.

I should be able to <u>find it</u>.
⟨clean the teeth⟩
I should be able to <u>clean the teeth</u>.

1. see the dentist this afternoon
2. help you
3. visit the dentist
4. get my teeth cleaned
5. find your office
6. meet with the patient
7. call soon
8. finish the treatment
9. meet you at two o'clock
10. find your dental clinic
11. find the exit
12. be on time for the appointment

Ⅴ．例文の下線部を以下の語句に置き換えなさい。

私は、それをみつけることができるはずです。
〈歯をクリーニングする〉
私は、歯をクリーニングすることができるはずです。

1. 今日の午後歯科医に診てもらう
2. あなたを手伝う
3. 歯医者に行く
4. 私の歯をクリーニングしてもらう
5. あなたの診療所をみつける
6. 患者に会う
7. もうすぐ電話する
8. 治療を終える
9. 2時にあなたに会う
10. あなたの歯科診療所をみつける
11. 出口をみつける
12. アポイントの時間どおりに行く

Chapter 4

Use of the telephone
Part IV: Questions about fees

How Much Will It Cost?

Aside from the charge for the initial examination, it is best not to discuss fees too much on the telephone. The fee varies considerably depending on the type of treatment. Tell the patient that he will be given a detailed estimate of treatment costs after the initial examination and before any work is done.

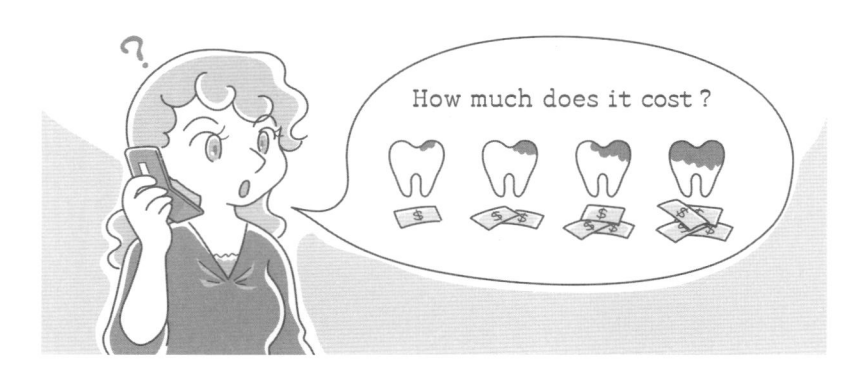

How much does it cost?

第 4 章

電話の応対
Ⅳ．診療費に関する質問

おいくらぐらいかかりますか？

　初診料以外は、診療費についてあまり電話で話さないのが一番よい。治療のタイプによって費用もかなり違ってくるからである。患者には、初診の後、何らかの治療がされる前に治療の詳しい見積りが渡される、と言っておくこと。

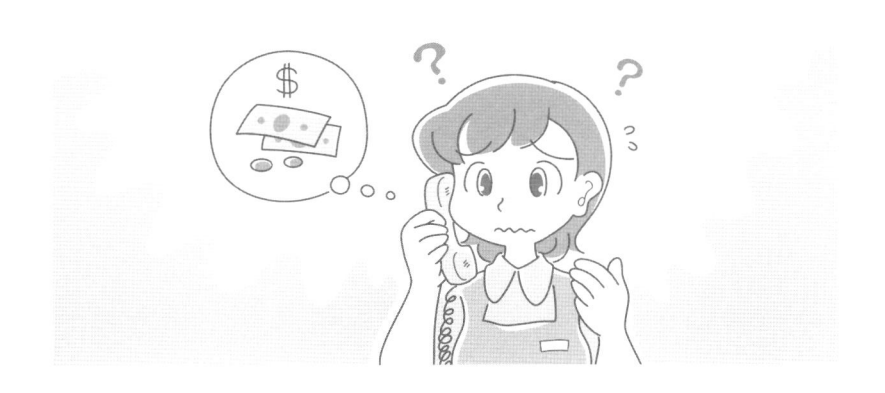

Situation: Mrs. Koch is calling to inquire about the cost of her dental treatment.

Ms. Fukuoka: Good morning. This is the Hayashi Dental Clinic. May I help you?

Mrs. Koch: My tooth is broken. Can you tell me how much it will cost to fix it?

Ms. Fukuoka: The fee varies considerably depending on what type of treatment is needed.

Mrs. Koch: It is a tooth in the back on the upper right side. How much does that one cost?

Ms. Fukuoka: It depends on whether it needs a crown or a filling. The doctor will have to examine it before he can determine what treatment is necessary.

Mrs. Koch: How much is the examination?

Ms. Fukuoka: The basic examination is seven thousand yen.

Mrs. Koch: I want a filling rather than a crown. How much does a filling cost?

Ms. Fukuoka: It depends on the size of the cavity. If the cavity is very large, it may be necessary to do a crown.

Mrs. Koch: Can I pay for it later?

Ms. Fukuoka: It is necessary to pay for the treatment when it is done.

Mrs. Koch: Well, I'll make an appointment later. Good bye.

Ms. Fukuoka: Good bye.

場面：カーチ夫人は、歯科治療の費用について尋ねるため電話をしている。

福岡さん：おはようございます。林歯科医院でございます。

カーチ夫人：私の歯が割れたのですが。治していただくのにいくらぐらいかかるか教えていただけますか。
福岡さん：どんなタイプの治療が必要かによって、費用もかなり違ってきます。
カーチ夫人：右上の奥歯なんですが、いくらかかりますか。

福岡さん：クラウンが必要か、充填が必要かによります。どんな治療が必要か決める前に、先生がその歯を調べなければなりません。
カーチ夫人：調べていただくのはいくらかかるでしょうか。
福岡さん：基本的な診査は7千円になっております。
カーチ夫人：私はクラウンよりも詰めていただきたいんです。充填はどのくらいですか。
福岡さん：それもむし歯の大きさによります。もしむし歯が大変大きければ、クラウンが必要になるかもしれません。
カーチ夫人：後でお支払いすることはできますか。
福岡さん：治療が終った時点でお支払いいただくことになっております。
カーチ夫人：じゃあ、また後で予約をします。さようなら。
福岡さん：失礼いたします。

Exercises

Ⅰ. Substitute the following expressions in the example sentence.

The fee varies considerably depending on the <u>type of treatment</u>.
⟨tooth⟩
The fee varies considerably depending on the <u>tooth</u>.

1. material
2. length of treatment
3. difficulty of the treatment
4. location of the tooth
5. laboratory expense
6. degree of difficulty
7. type of material
8. type of tooth
9. material used
10. metal
11. value of the metal
12. time required

Ⅱ. Substitute the following expressions in the example sentence.

He inquired about the cost of <u>treatment</u>.
⟨the crown⟩
He inquired about the cost of <u>the crown</u>.

練習問題

Ⅰ．例文の下線部を以下の語句に置き換えなさい。

治療のタイプによって、費用もかなり違ってくる。
〈歯〉
歯によって、費用もかなり違ってくる。

 1．材料
 2．治療の長さ
 3．治療の難しさ
 4．歯の位置
 5．技工料
 6．難易度
 7．材料のタイプ
 8．歯のタイプ
 9．使われる材料
10．金属
11．金属の値打ち
12．所要時間

Ⅱ．例文の下線部を以下の語句に置き換えなさい。

彼は治療の費用について尋ねた。
〈クラウン〉
彼はクラウンの費用について尋ねた。

1. the filling
2. a cleaning
3. a porcelain crown
4. a new denture
5. his dental treatment
6. dental services
7. cleaning his teeth
8. the toothbrush
9. the inlay
10. an amalgam restoration
11. an insurance crown
12. insurance treatment

Ⅲ. Substitute the following expressions in the example sentence.

Tell the patient that he will be given a detailed estimate.
⟨a complete examination⟩
Tell the patient that he will be given a complete examination.

1. a new crown
2. directions to the office
3. the X-rays
4. a letter of introduction
5. a new denture
6. time to think about the proposed treatment
7. my telephone number
8. some antibiotics

1. 充填
2. クリーニング
3. ポーセレンクラウン
4. 新しい義歯
5. 彼の歯科治療
6. 歯科治療
7. 歯のクリーニング
8. 歯ブラシ
9. インレー
10. アマルガム修復物
11. 保険でできるクラウン
12. 保険治療

Ⅲ. 例文の下線部を以下の語句に置き換えなさい。

<u>詳しい見積り</u>が渡されると、患者に言っておくこと。
〈徹底的な診査〉
<u>徹底的な診査</u>がされると、患者に言っておくこと。

1. 新しいクラウン
2. 診療所への道順
3. エックス線写真
4. 紹介状
5. 新しい義歯
6. 計画された治療について考える時間
7. 私の電話番号
8. 抗生物質

9. a new porcelain crown
10. a pain killer
11. a copy of the dental records
12. his X-rays

Ⅳ. Substitute the following expressions in the example sentence.

How much will it cost to <u>fix the tooth</u>?
〈repair the denture〉
How much will it cost to <u>repair the denture</u>?

1. examine the teeth
2. replace the crown
3. clean the teeth
4. restore my teeth
5. have that filling replaced
6. consult with the dentist
7. have the cleaning done
8. have a new set of dentures made
9. replace the porcelain crown
10. extract the tooth
11. do the root canal treatment
12. have X-rays taken

9. 新しいポーセレンクラウン
10. 痛みどめ
11. 歯科記録のコピー
12. 彼のエックス線写真

Ⅳ．例文の下線部を以下の語句に置き換えなさい。

その歯を治すのに、いくらかかるでしょうか。
〈その義歯を修理する〉
その義歯を修理するのに、いくらかかるでしょうか。

1. その歯を調べる
2. そのクラウンを取りかえる
3. その歯をクリーニングする
4. 私の歯を修復する
5. その充填を取りかえてもらう
6. 歯医者さんに相談する
7. クリーニングをしてもらう
8. 新しい義歯を一式作ってもらう
9. そのポーセレンクラウンを取りかえてもらう
10. その歯を抜く
11. 根管治療をする
12. エックス線写真を撮ってもらう

V. Substitute the following expressions in the example dialogue.

— How much is the <u>examination</u>?
— It is <u>seven thousand</u> yen.
⟨treatment/fifteen thousand⟩
— How much is the <u>treatment</u>?
— It is <u>fifteen thousand</u> yen.

1. examination/eight hundred
2. crown/eighty thousand
3. inlay/ten thousand
4. cleaning/two thousand five hundred
5. entire treatment/five hundred thousand
6. root canal treatment/twenty thousand
7. initial examination/two thousand
8. denture/one hundred thousand
9. porcelain crown/one hundred thousand
10. interproximal brush/two hundred
11. plastic filling/eight thousand
12. bridge/two hundred thousand

Ⅴ．例にあげた対話の下線部を以下の語句に置き換えなさい。

－<u>診査</u>はいくらですか。
－<u>7千</u>円です。
〈治療／1万5千円〉
－<u>治療</u>はいくらですか。
－<u>1万5千</u>円です。

1. 診査／8百
2. クラウン／8万
3. インレー／1万
4. クリーニング／2千5百
5. 全部の治療／50万
6. 根管治療／2万
7. 初診／2千
8. 義歯／10万
9. ポーセレンクラウン／10万
10. 歯間ブラシ／2百
11. プラスチックの充填／8千
12. ブリッジ／20万

Chapter 5

Use of the telephone
Part V: Cancellation of an appointment

I Am Too Busy to Keep My Appointment This Afternoon.

Appointment cancellations can be very costly for the dentist in terms of lost working time. People who cancel appointments will often cancel habitually. They should be told how important it is to keep their appointments.

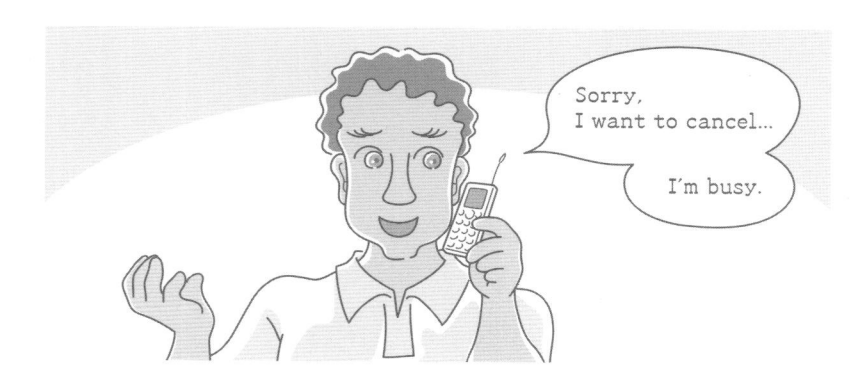

Sorry, I want to cancel...

I'm busy.

第 5 章

電話の応対
V. アポイントのキャンセル

とても忙しくて、午後の予約時間に行けないんですが

　アポイントのキャンセルは、診療時間が無駄になるという意味で、歯科医にとって大変高いものにつく場合もある。アポイントをキャンセルする人々はキャンセルの常習であることも多い。このような人たちには、アポイントを守ることがいかに大切であるか言わなければならない。

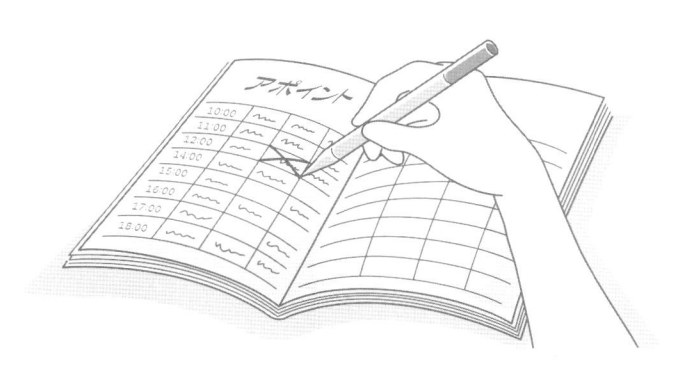

Situation: Mr. Delan, a Frenchman, is calling to cancel an appointment.

Ms. Fukuoka: Hello. This is the Hayashi Dental Clinic. May I help you?
Mr. Delan: This is Charles Delan. I am too busy to keep my appointment this afternoon. Can you schedule it another time?
Ms. Fukuoka: The doctor has reserved that time for you and is expecting you at two o'clock.
Mr. Delan: But I am a very busy man.
Ms. Fukuoka: The doctor is also quite busy. If the appointment is broken at this time, it will probably be impossible to fill it with another patient. That leaves the time wasted by the entire staff here.
Mr. Delan: But my wife wanted me to go shopping with her this afternoon.
Ms. Fukuoka: Can't you do that another time?
Mr. Delan: I will have to ask her.
Ms. Fukuoka: It is very important for you not to break appointments at the last minute like this.
Mr. Delan: OK. I will try to be there at two. Good bye.
Ms. Fukuoka: Good bye.

場面：フランス人のデラン氏は、アポイントをキャンセルするために電話をしている。

福岡さん：もしもし。林歯科医院でございます。

デラン氏：こちらはチャールズ・デランです。とても忙しくて、今日の午後の予約時間に行けないのですが、別の時に変えていただけますか。

福岡さん：先生は、その時間をデランさんのために取って、2時においでになるのをお待ちしているのですが。

デラン氏：でも、私はとても忙しいんですよ。

福岡さん：先生も大変忙しいんです。もし今回の予約を破られると、他の患者さんにその時間来ていただくのも多分無理でしょう。そうすると、こちらのスタッフ全員に無駄な時間ができてしまいます。

デラン氏：でも、妻が今日の午後一緒に買い物についてきてほしいと言っていましてね。

福岡さん：別の時にしていただけませんか。

デラン氏：妻に聞かないとね。

福岡さん：こんなに直前に、予約を破ることがないようにしていただくことが大切です。

デラン氏：わかりました。2時に行くようにしましょう。さようなら。

福岡さん：失礼いたします。

Exercises

I. Substitute the following expressions in the example sentence.

I am too busy to <u>keep my appointment this afternoon</u>.
⟨brush my teeth⟩
I am too busy to <u>brush my teeth</u>.

1. visit the dentist
2. take care of my teeth
3. reschedule the appointment
4. floss my teeth
5. clean my teeth
6. do the filling
7. come to your office
8. see my dentist
9. brush my children's teeth
10. floss my child's teeth
11. take my husband to the dentist
12. clean my teeth properly

II. Substitute the following expressions in the example sentence.

The doctor is expecting <u>you</u>.
⟨to see you⟩
The doctor is expecting <u>to see you</u>.

練習問題

Ⅰ．例文の下線部を以下の語句に置き換えなさい。

とても忙しくて、今日の午後の予約時間に行けません。
〈歯を磨く〉
とても忙しくて、歯を磨けません。

1. 歯医者に行く
2. 歯の手入れをする
3. 予約を変更する
4. 歯をフロッシングする
5. 歯をきれいにする
6. 充填をする
7. あなたの診療所に行く
8. 私の歯医者に診てもらう
9. 子どもたちの歯を磨く
10. 子どもの歯をフロッシングする
11. 夫を歯医者に連れていく
12. きちんと歯を磨く

Ⅱ．例文の下線部を以下の語句に置き換えなさい。

先生はあなたをお待ちしています。
〈あなたを診ること〉
先生はあなたを診るのを期待しています。

1. a phone call
2. to receive a phone call
3. to receive a phone call from you
4. a patient
5. to see a patient
6. to see a patient from Africa
7. a letter
8. to receive a letter
9. to receive a letter from the insurance company
10. a delivery
11. to receive a delivery
12. to receive a delivery of dental floss

Ⅲ. Substitute the following expressions in the example sentence.

My wife wanted me to go shopping with her.
⟨stop smoking⟩
My wife wanted me to stop smoking.

1. see the dentist
2. reschedule the appointment
3. have her teeth cleaned
4. cancel the appointment
5. confirm the appointment
6. change the appointment time
7. schedule an appointment
8. make an appointment with the hygienist

1. 電話
2. 電話がかかってくること
3. あなたから電話がかかってくること
4. 患者
5. 患者と会うこと
6. アフリカからの患者を診ること
7. 手紙
8. 手紙を受け取ること
9. 保険会社から手紙を受け取ること
10. 配達
11. 配達を受け取ること
12. 歯科用フロスの配達を受け取ること

Ⅲ．例文の下線部を以下の語句に置き換えなさい。

妻は、私に一緒に買い物に行ってほしかった。
〈たばこをやめる〉
妻は、私にたばこをやめてほしかった。

1. 歯医者に行く
2. 予約を変更する
3. 私の歯をクリーニングする
4. 予約をキャンセルする
5. 予約を確認する
6. 予約時間を変更する
7. 予約を取る
8. 歯科衛生士との予約を取る

9. brush my teeth
10. pay my dental bill
11. call the dentist
12. visit the doctor

Ⅳ. Substitute the following expressions in the example sentence.

I will try to be there <u>at two</u>.
⟨soon⟩
I will try to be there <u>soon</u>.

1. as soon as possible
2. on time
3. by two o'clock
4. at the correct time
5. in the evening
6. early
7. earlier than before
8. in one hour
9. before you arrive
10. tomorrow
11. tomorrow evening
12. Wednesday at three o'clock

9. 私の歯を磨く
10. 歯科費用を支払う
11. 歯医者に電話する
12. 医者に行く

Ⅳ．例文の下線部を以下の語句に置き換えなさい。

2時にそこに行くようにしましょう。
〈すぐに〉
すぐにそこに行くようにしましょう。

1. できるだけすぐに
2. 時間どおりに
3. 2時までに
4. 正確な時間に
5. 夜に
6. 早くに
7. 前より早く
8. 1時間で
9. あなたが着く前に
10. 明日
11. 明日の夜
12. 水曜日3時に

V. Substitute the following expressions in the example sentence.

It will probably be impossible to save that tooth.
〈clean his teeth〉
It will probably be impossible to clean his teeth.

1. be on time
2. complete treatment today
3. clean the teeth in one visit
4. finish the work on time
5. find a better dentist
6. place a crown on that tooth
7. treat that periodontal condition
8. get an appointment for tomorrow
9. clean your teeth today
10. arrive on time
11. find a better hygienist
12. make a more beautiful crown

Ⅴ．例文の下線部を以下の語句に置き換えなさい。

その歯を残すのはたぶん無理でしょう。
〈彼の歯をクリーニングする〉
彼の歯をクリーニングするのはたぶん無理でしょう。

1. 時間を守る
2. 今日治療を終える
3. 1回の来院で歯をクリーニングする
4. 時間どおりにその仕事を終える
5. もっとよい歯医者をみつける
6. その歯にクラウンを装着する
7. その歯周状態を治療する
8. 明日の予約を取る
9. 今日歯をクリーニングする
10. 時間どおりに着く
11. もっとよい歯科衛生士をみつける
12. もっと美しいクラウンを作る

Chapter 6

Use of the telephone
Part Ⅵ : A call for the doctor

May I Talk with the Doctor?

You may often receive calls from patients wishing to talk with the doctor directly. If he is treating a patient, it may be very difficult for him to come to the phone. He should not be interrupted unless absolutely necessary when he is with a patient. It is important to tell the caller that the doctor is with a patient and he will return the call later.

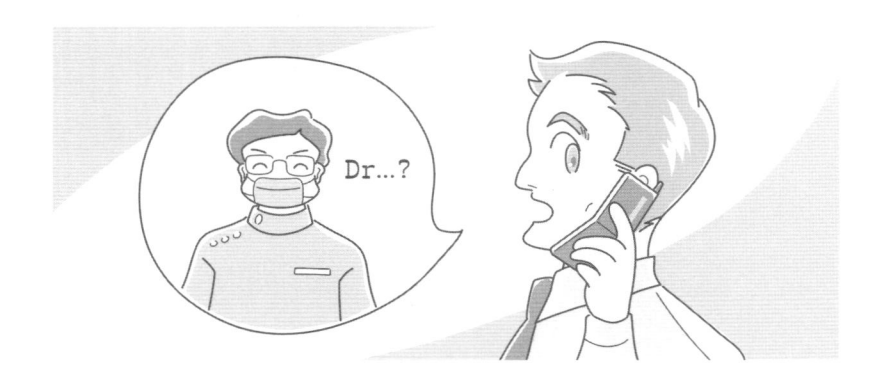

第 6 章

電話の応対
Ⅵ. 医師への電話

先生とお話できますか？

　先生と直接話したいという電話をよく患者から受けることがあるかもしれない。もし患者を治療中なら、電話口に出るのは非常に難しいであろう。医師が治療中は、絶対に必要な時以外、邪魔してはいけない。電話をかけた人には、今患者を診ているので後でこちらから電話をすると言うことが大切である。

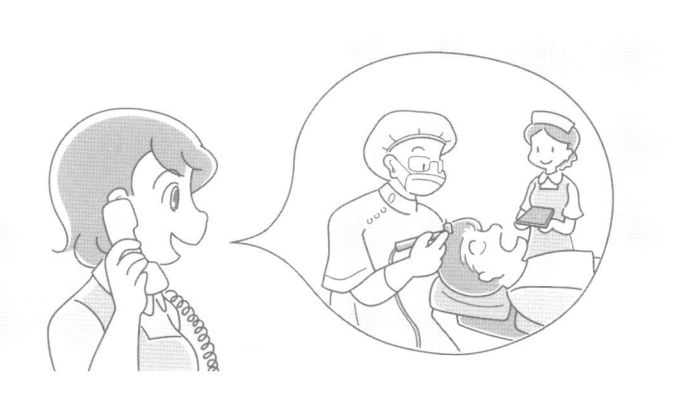

Situation: Mr. Burke is calling the doctor to discuss his daughter's treatment. The doctor is with a patient and cannot come to the phone.

Ms. Fukuoka: Good afternoon. This is the Hayashi Dental Clinic. May I help you?

Mr. Burke: This is Frank Burke. May I speak with Dr. Hayashi?

Ms. Fukuoka: I am sorry. He is with a patient now and cannot come to the phone.

Mr. Burke: I wanted to talk about my daughter's braces. When will he be available?

Ms. Fukuoka: His schedule is very busy but he should be able to call you later in the afternoon.

Mr. Burke: That would be fine. Please have him call me at the office.

Ms. Fukuoka: Certainly. I will have him call as soon as possible.

Mr. Burke: It is not urgent, but I would like to talk with him soon if possible. You have my number, don't you?

Ms. Fukuoka: Yes. It is in your chart.

Mr. Burke: I will be expecting his call. Good bye.

Ms. Fukuoka: Good bye.

場面：バーク氏は、娘の治療について相談するため電話をしている。医師は患者を診ていて、電話に出ることができない。

福岡さん：はい。林歯科医院でございます。

バーク氏：こちらはフランク・バークです。先生とお話できますか。

福岡さん：申し訳ございません。先生は、ただいま患者さんを診ておりまして、電話に出られませんが。

バーク氏：娘の矯正装置についてお話したかったんですがね。いつお手すきになりますか。

福岡さん：先生の予定は大変忙しいのですが、後ほど午後にお電話できるはずです。

バーク氏：それでけっこうです。私の事務所の方にお電話くださるようお伝えください。

福岡さん：かしこまりました。できるだけすぐに電話するように申します。

バーク氏：緊急ではないんですが、できればすぐに先生とお話したいので。私の電話番号はおわかりになりますね。

福岡さん：はい。カルテに入っております。

バーク氏：じゃあ、お電話お待ちしています。さようなら。

福岡さん：失礼いたします。

Exercises

Ⅰ. Substitute the following expressions in the example sentence.

It is difficult for the doctor to <u>come to the phone</u>.
⟨complete the work today⟩
It is difficult for the doctor to <u>complete the work today</u>.

1. see you now
2. come to the waiting room
3. finish the work today
4. see two patients at the same time
5. interrupt treatment to come to the phone
6. work on Sunday
7. treat children
8. take X-rays of uncooperative children
9. finish the root canal treatment in one day
10. see you today
11. talk while he is working
12. delay treatment on the patients currently waiting

Ⅱ. Substitute the following expressions in the example sentence.

He should not be <u>interrupted</u>.
⟨scolded⟩
He should not be <u>scolded</u>.

練習問題

Ⅰ．例文の下線部を以下の語句に置き換えなさい。

医師が電話に出るのは難しい。
〈今日その仕事を終える〉
医師が今日その仕事を終えるのは難しい。

1. 今あなたに会う
2. 待合室に来る
3. 今日その仕事を終える
4. 同時に2人の患者を診る
5. 電話口に来るために治療を中断する
6. 日曜日に働く
7. 子どもの治療をする
8. 協力的でない子どものエックス線写真を撮る
9. 1日で根管治療を終える
10. 今日あなたに会う
11. 働きながら話す
12. 今待っている患者の治療を延期する

Ⅱ．例文の下線部を以下の語句に置き換えなさい。

彼を邪魔してはいけない。
〈叱る〉
彼を叱ってはいけない。

1. interrupted too often
2. reappointed
3. told to leave the office
4. appointed if the doctor is unavailable
5. rescheduled
6. given another appointment
7. discouraged when his brushing is inadequate
8. taken to the dentist if he has the flu
9. interrupted while treating a patient
10. treated badly
11. given brushing instructions now
12. denied treatment

Ⅲ. Substitute the following expressions in the example dialogue.

− May I speak with the doctor?
− I am sorry. He is <u>with a patient</u>.
⟨busy⟩
− May I speak with the doctor?
− I am sorry. He is <u>busy</u>.

1. out of the office
2. out to lunch
3. talking with a patient
4. on the phone
5. not here
6. seeing a patient

1. 何度も中断する
2. 再予約する
3. （彼に）診療所から出ていくように言う
4. 歯科医が無理なのに（彼に）アポイントを取る
5. 予約し直す
6. （彼に）またアポイントを取ってあげる
7. ブラッシングが適切でなくてもやる気をなくさせる
8. 彼がインフルエンザにかかっていたら歯医者につれてくる
9. （彼が）患者を治療中邪魔する
10. ひどい扱いをする
11. 今、歯ブラシ指導をする
12. 治療するのを拒否する

Ⅲ．例にあげた対話の下線部を以下の語句に置き換えなさい。

－先生とお話できますか。
－申し訳ございません。先生は患者を診ています。
〈忙しい〉
－先生とお話できますか。
－申し訳ございません。先生は忙しいです。

1. 外出しています
2. 昼食に出ています
3. 患者と話しています
4. 電話中です
5. ここにおりません
6. 患者を診ています

7. busy now

8. working in the laboratory

9. outside

10. on vacation

11. out of town

12. at a dental convention

Ⅳ. Substitute the following expressions in the example sentence.

Please have the doctor <u>call me at the office</u>.
⟨make a new denture⟩
Please have the doctor <u>make a new denture</u>.

1. call me back
2. give me a phone call
3. clean my teeth
4. examine my teeth
5. check the hygienist's work
6. place an amalgam filling
7. give me some medicine
8. check my teeth
9. take an X-ray
10. review my records
11. look at the X-ray
12. return to the office

7. 今忙しい
8. ラボで働いております
9. 外に出ております
10. 休暇中です
11. 町から出ております
12. 歯科学会に行っております

Ⅳ．例文の下線部を以下の語句に置き換えなさい。

先生に私の事務所の方に電話するように伝えてください。
〈新しい義歯を作る〉
先生に新しい義歯を作るように伝えてください。

1. 私に電話をかけ直す
2. 私に電話をする
3. 私の歯をクリーニングする
4. 私の歯を調べる
5. 歯科衛生士の仕事をチェックする
6. アマルガム充填を装着する
7. 私に薬を渡す
8. 私の歯をチェックする
9. エックス線写真を撮る
10. 私の記録をもう一度見る
11. そのエックス線写真を見る
12. 診療所に戻る

V. Substitute the following expressions in the example sentence.

I will have him <u>call</u> as soon as possible.
⟨see you⟩
I will have him <u>see you</u> as soon as possible.

1. call you
2. contact you
3. give you a prescription
4. repair the denture
5. clean your teeth
6. make an appointment
7. call for an appointment
8. make a new partial denture
9. send the bill to the company
10. fill out the insurance form
11. write an estimate
12. make a treatment plan

Ⅴ．例文の下線部を以下の語句に置き換えなさい。

できるだけすぐに電話するように申します。
〈あなたに会う〉
できるだけすぐにあなたに会うように申します。

1. あなたに電話する
2. あなたに連絡する
3. あなたに処方箋を渡す
4. 義歯を修理する
5. あなたの歯をクリーニングする
6. アポイントを取る
7. アポイントのために電話をする
8. 新しい部分義歯を作る
9. 請求書を会社に送る
10. 保険の用紙に書き入れる
11. 見積りを書く
12. 治療計画を立てる

Chapter 7

Greeting the patient

I Am Afraid It Has Been a Long Time Since My Last Checkup.

Every patient should be made to feel welcome when he comes to the office, whether it is his first visit or if he has been a patient for several years. It is best not to immediately inquire about the teeth since this might make the patient think that his only value to you is in his teeth. Rather, you might consider some general inquiry into his health or about his family.

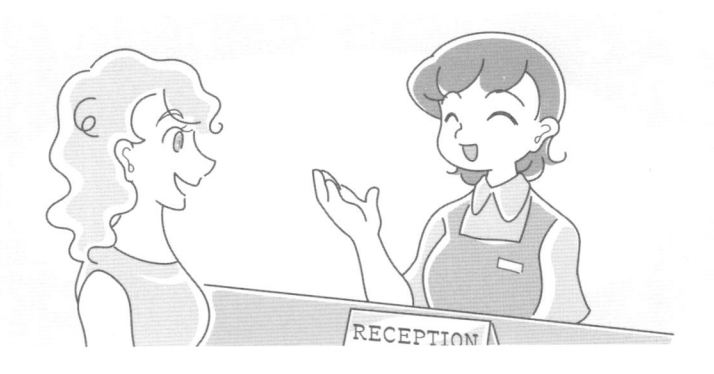

第 7 章

患者へのあいさつ

この前の検診からずいぶんたったようですね

　患者が来院する時は、初めての人も、数年来の患者であっても、自分が喜んで迎えられていると感じさせなければならない。すぐに歯について質問しないのがよい。というのは、それで患者は、あなたにとって大切なことは彼の歯だけだと思うかもしれないからである。それよりむしろ、患者の健康や家族について一般的な質問をすることを考えた方が良いだろう。

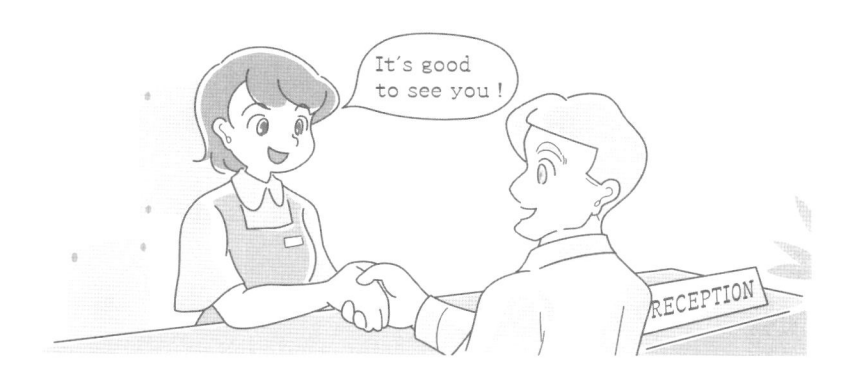

It's good to see you!

Situation: Mr. Baker, an American diplomat, is returning to the clinic for a routine checkup. He has been a patient here for several years.

Ms. Wakai: Hello Mr. Baker. It is good to see you.
Mr. Baker: Thank you. I am afraid it has been a long time since my last checkup.
Ms. Wakai: How have you been lately?
Mr. Baker: Well I have been quite busy of late due to the trade negotiations. You know what they say in Japanese — "bimbo hima nashi."
Ms. Wakai: You are getting pretty good at Japanese. How do you say that in English?
Mr. Baker: We poor folk never have any free time.
Ms. Wakai: The doctor will be ready to see you in a few minutes.
Mr. Baker: Fine.
Ms. Wakai: Do you have any special problem with your teeth or is this appointment just for a checkup?
Mr. Baker: Just a checkup and cleaning. I think that my teeth are fine.
Ms. Wakai: That's good. Please have a seat. The doctor will be with you soon.
Mr. Baker: Thank you.

場面：アメリカ人外交官、ベイカー氏は定期検診のために再来院。彼は数年来ずっとここの患者である。

若井さん：ベイカーさん、こんにちは。よくいらっしゃいました。
ベイカー氏：ありがとう。この前の検診からずいぶんたったようですね。
若井さん：最近はどうしていらっしゃいますか。
ベイカー氏：ええ。最近、通商交渉のためにかなり忙しくしているんです。日本語でも言うでしょう。貧乏暇なしってね。
若井さん：日本語が大変お上手になられていますね。それは、英語でどう言うのですか。
ベイカー氏：We poor folks never have any free time.
若井さん：先生は2〜3分で診察できます。
ベイカー氏：わかりました。
若井さん：歯に特に何か問題がありますか。それとも検診だけの予約でしょうか。
ベイカー氏：検診とクリーニングだけです。歯は大丈夫だと思います。
若井さん：それはよかったですね。どうぞおかけください。先生はすぐに参りますから。
ベイカー氏：ありがとう。

Exercises

I. Substitute the following expressions in the example sentence.

He has been a patient here <u>for several years</u>.
⟨for two years⟩
He has been a patient here <u>for two years</u>.

1. for some time
2. for a long time
3. as long as I can remember
4. since he came to Osaka
5. recently
6. for only a few weeks
7. for three months
8. since the doctor first began practicing
9. since he was a child
10. for eight years
11. for about a year
12. for about two years

II. Substitute the following expressions in the example sentence.

I am afraid it has been a long time since <u>my last checkup</u>.
⟨I came to your clinic⟩
I am afraid it has been a long time since <u>I came to your clinic</u>.

練習問題

Ⅰ．例文の下線部を以下の語句に置き換えなさい。

彼は、数年来ずっとここの患者である。
〈2年間〉
彼は、2年間ずっとここの患者である。

1. しばらくの間
2. 長い間
3. 私が覚えている限り
4. 彼が大阪に来て以来
5. 最近
6. 2～3週間の間だけ
7. 3ヵ月
8. 歯科医が開業してから
9. 子どもの時から
10. 8年間
11. 約1年間
12. 約2年間

Ⅱ．例文の下線部を、以下の語句に置き換えなさい。

この前の検診からずいぶんたったようですね。
〈あなたの診療所に来る〉
あなたの診療所に来てからずいぶんたったようですね。

1. my last cleaning appointment
2. I brushed my teeth
3. he visited the dentist
4. she saw a dentist
5. I had any dental treatment
6. I brushed my son's teeth
7. he saw a hygienist
8. he took care of his teeth
9. I had X-rays taken
10. I had the filling replaced
11. she cleaned my teeth
12. I visited a doctor

Ⅲ. Substitute the following expressions in the example dialogue.

―How do you say, "<u>bimbo hima nashi</u>" in English?
―<u>We poor folk never have any free time.</u>
⟨"haisha" /dentist⟩
―How do you say, "<u>haisha</u>" in English?
―<u>Dentist</u>.

1. "shikon" /root
2. "konkan chiryo" /root canal treatment
3. "shikadaigaku" /Dental University
4. "shikou" /plaque
5. "bimbo yusuri" /nervous shaking of the body
6. "watashi uso tsukanai" /I don't speak with a forked tongue

1. この前のクリーニング・アポイント
2. 私が歯を磨いた
3. 彼が歯医者に行った
4. 彼女が歯医者に診てもらった
5. 私が歯科治療を受けた
6. 私が息子の歯を磨いた
7. 彼が歯科衛生士に診てもらった
8. 彼が自分の歯の手入れをした
9. 私の歯のエックス線写真を撮る
10. 私の充填物を取りかえた
11. 彼女が私の歯をクリーニングした
12. 私がお医者さんに行った

Ⅲ. 例にあげた対話の下線部を以下の語句に置き換えなさい。

－「貧乏暇なし」は英語でどう言うのですか。
－we poor folks never have any free time.
〈歯医者〉
－「歯医者」は英語でどう言うのですか。
－Dentist.

1. 歯根
2. 根管治療
3. 歯科大学
4. プラーク
5. 貧乏ゆすり
6. 私うそつかない

7. "shikan burashi" /interproximal brush
8. "gakubuchi kinkan" /window crown
9. "kinba" /gold tooth
10. "hayaoki wa sanmon no toku" /the early bird gets the worm
11. "ha ga ukuyou na oseji" /obvious flattery
12. "ireba" /denture

Ⅳ. Substitute the following expressions in the example sentence.

Do you have any special problem with your <u>teeth</u>?
〈health〉
Do you have any special problem with your <u>health</u>?

1. dental health
2. dentures
3. occlusion
4. gums
5. crown
6. partial denture
7. teeth or gums
8. heart
9. splint
10. fillings
11. brushing and flossing
12. dental treatment

7. 歯間ブラシ
8. 額縁金冠
9. 金歯
10. 早起きは三文の得
11. 歯が浮くようなお世辞
12. 入れ歯

Ⅳ．例文の下線部を以下の語句に置き換えなさい。

あなたの歯に特に何か問題がありますか。
〈健康〉
あなたの健康に特に何か問題がありますか。

1. 歯の健康
2. 入れ歯
3. 咬合
4. 歯ぐき
5. クラウン
6. 部分義歯
7. 歯または歯ぐき
8. 心臓
9. スプリント
10. 充填物
11. ブラッシングとフロッシング
12. 歯科治療

Ⅴ. Substitute the following expressions in the example dialogue.

− Please have a seat. The doctor will <u>see you</u> in about five minutes.
− Thank you.
〈examine you〉
− Please have a seat. The doctor will <u>examine you</u> in about five minutes.
− Thank you.

1. examine your teeth
2. start work
3. start your examination
4. begin work on the crown
5. clean your teeth
6. give you the estimate
7. talk about the treatment plan
8. look at the X-rays
9. go over your treatment plan
10. begin your consultation
11. start treatment
12. begin your treatment

Ⅴ．例にあげた対話の下線部を以下の語句に置き換えなさい。

－どうぞ、お掛けください。先生は5分ぐらいで<u>あなたを診</u>ます。

－ありがとう。
〈あなたを診察する〉
－どうぞ、お掛けください。先生は5分ぐらいで<u>あなたを診察し</u>ます。
－ありがとう。

 1. あなたの歯を調べる
 2. 仕事を始める
 3. あなたの診察を始める
 4. クラウンの仕事を始める
 5. あなたの歯をクリーニングする
 6. あなたに見積りを渡す
 7. 治療計画について話す
 8. エックス線写真を見る
 9. あなたの治療計画を検討する
10. あなたの相談に応じる（始める）
11. 治療を始める
12. あなたの治療を始める

Chapter 8

Preparing the forms for foreign dental insurance

Does The Dentist Accept This Insurance?

Many foreigners in Japan have dental insurance from foreign insurance companies. This insurance is considerably different from Japanese National Health Insurance. The patient should pay for his treatment at the time it is done and the insurance company will reimburse him later. The patient usually receives from the insurance company 50 to 70% of the amount he pays the dentist.

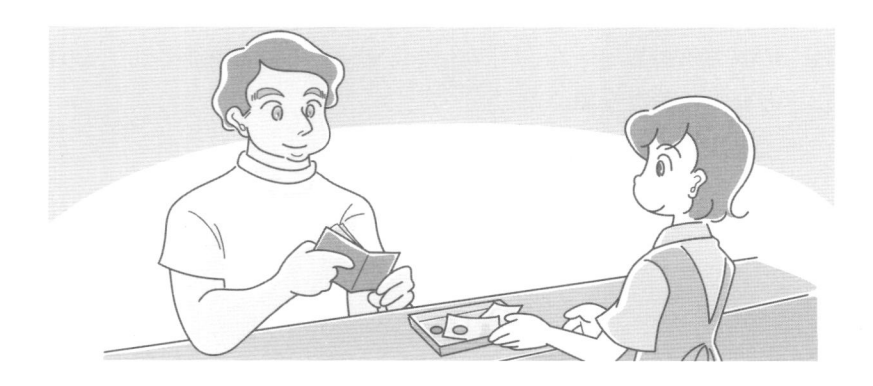

第 8 章

外国の保険の用紙に書き入れる

先生はこの保険を受けていらっしゃいますか？

　日本にいる外国人の多くは外国の保険会社の歯科保険を持っている。この保険は日本の健康保険とかなり違う。患者は治療が終った時点でその治療費を払い、保険会社が後で患者に払い戻すことになっている。患者は、歯科医に支払った額の50％から70％を、保険会社から受け取るのが普通である。

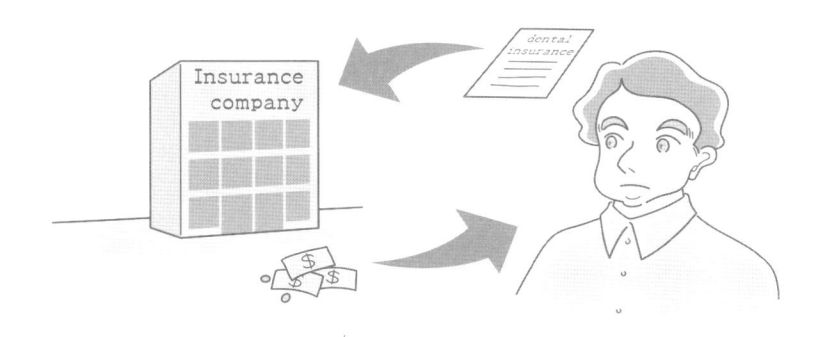

Situation: Mr. Burton is a Frenchman employed by a large multinational company. His company provides dental insurance for him through an American insurance company. The receptionist is discussing the use of this insurance.

Mr. Burton: I would like to have my dental treatment done here. Does the dentist accept this insurance? (He shows the forms to the receptionist.)

Ms. Umeda: Yes. We often have patients who use this type of dental insurance.

Mr. Burton: That's good.

Ms. Umeda: However, it is necessary to have you pay for the treatment as it is done. The dentist will then fill out the forms and the insurance company will reimburse you directly.

Mr. Burton: I understand. Usually I get back about 70% of the total bill.

Ms. Umeda: Each company is different. Some pay more than others.

Mr. Burton: Do you have any trouble with this type of insurance?

Ms. Umeda: None, yet. Sometimes they ask us to send X-rays. The mail takes a long time.

Mr. Burton: How long will it take to get back the money?

Ms. Umeda: Most of our patients are reimbursed in two to three months.

Mr. Burton: That's good. I need the money. Even foreigners are troubled by the high value of the yen.

場面：バートン氏は大きな多国籍企業に勤めるフランス人である。彼の会社は、アメリカの保険会社を通じて、彼の歯科保険に入っている。受付がこの保険の使用について相談している。

バートン氏：こちらで歯科治療を受けたいのですが、先生はこの保険を受付けていらっしゃいますか。（受付にその用紙を見せる。）
梅田さん：はい。こちらでは、このような歯科保険をお使いになる患者さんがよくいらっしゃいます。
バートン氏：それはよかった。
梅田さん：ですけれど、治療が終った時に患者さんにお支払いいただく必要があります。それから先生がその用紙に書き入れて、保険会社が患者さんに直接払い戻すことになっています。
バートン氏：ええ、知っています。普通は合計金額の70％を返してもらっています。
梅田さん：それぞれ会社によって違います。他より多く支払うところもありますし。
バートン氏：このような保険で何か困ることがありますか。
梅田さん：いいえ、ぜんぜんありません。時々、エックス線写真を送るように頼まれますが、郵便は時間がかかります。
バートン氏：お金を返してもらうのにどのくらいかかるでしょうか。
梅田さん：ここの患者さんはほとんど、2～3ヵ月で払い戻しを受けていらっしゃいます。
バートン氏：それはよかった。お金がいるんですよ。外国人だって円高で困っていますから。

Exercises

I. Substitute the following expressions in the example sentence.

<u>Teeth</u> are different from <u>bones</u>.
⟨plaque/food debris⟩
<u>Plaque</u> is different from <u>food debris</u>.

1. root canal treatment/a filling
2. porcelain/plastic
3. composite resin/amalgam
4. my teeth/your teeth
5. hygienists/dentists
6. insurance treatment/fee for service treatment
7. cleaning by a hygienist/brushing your own teeth
8. molars/incisors
9. dental treatment/medical treatment
10. premolars/molars
11. crowns/inlays
12. a crown/an amalgam filling

II. Substitute the following expressions in the example sentence.

I would like to <u>have my dental treatment done here</u>.
⟨see a film on brushing⟩
I would like to <u>see a film on brushing</u>.

練習問題

Ⅰ．例文の下線部を以下の語句に置き換えなさい。

<u>歯</u>は<u>骨</u>とは違う。
〈プラーク／食べかす〉
<u>プラーク</u>は<u>食べかす</u>とは違う。

1. 根管治療／充填
2. ポーセレン／プラスチック
3. コンポジットレジン／アマルガム
4. 私の歯／あなたの歯
5. 歯科衛生士／歯科医
6. 保険治療／自由診療
7. 歯科衛生士によるクリーニング／自分自身で歯を磨くこと
8. 臼歯／切歯
9. 歯科治療／医科治療
10. 小臼歯／臼歯
11. クラウン／インレー
12. クラウン／アマルガム充填

Ⅱ．例文の下線部を以下の語句に置き換えなさい。

<u>こちらで歯科治療を受け</u>たいです。
〈ブラッシングについての映画を見る〉
<u>ブラッシングについての映画を見</u>たいです。

1. have my teeth cleaned
2. keep my teeth
3. prevent periodontal disease
4. have a cleaning
5. avoid tooth decay
6. have a beautiful smile
7. see the dentist
8. pay my bill
9. have my treatment completed
10. rinse my mouth
11. have a porcelain-fused-to-metal bridge
12. have a set of dentures

Ⅲ. Substitute the following expressions in the example sentence.

Do you have trouble with <u>this type of insurance</u>?
⟨your teeth⟩
Do you have trouble with <u>your teeth</u>?

1. your dentures
2. your gums
3. the partial denture
4. the crown
5. the interproximal brush
6. brushing
7. gum disease
8. periodontal disease

1. 私の歯をクリーニングしてもらう
2. ずっと自分の歯でいる
3. 歯周病を予防する
4. クリーニングを受ける
5. むし歯を避ける
6. 美しい笑顔をもつ
7. 歯医者に診てもらう
8. 治療費を払う
9. 私の治療を終えてもらう
10. 私の口をゆすぐ
11. ポーセレン焼き付金属ブリッジをしてもらう
12. 義歯一式をもらう

Ⅲ．例文の下線部を以下の語句に置き換えなさい。

<u>このような保険</u>で困ることがありますか。
〈あなたの歯〉
<u>あなたの歯</u>で困ることがありますか。

1. 義歯
2. あなたの歯ぐき
3. 部分義歯
4. クラウン
5. 歯間ブラシ
6. ブラッシング
7. 歯ぐきの病気
8. 歯周病

9. flossing
10. tooth decay
11. dental caries
12. plaque

Ⅳ. Substitute the following expressions in the example sentence.

How long will it take to <u>receive my reimbursement</u>?
⟨clean my teeth⟩
How long will it take to <u>clean my teeth</u>?

1. finish the treatment
2. complete my treatment
3. finish that crown
4. get an appointment
5. prepare the teeth
6. learn how to brush
7. reschedule the appointment
8. remove the plaque
9. complete that amalgam filling
10. make the crown
11. restore my teeth
12. receive money from the insurance company

9. フロッシング
10. むし歯
11. う蝕
12. プラーク

Ⅳ．例文の下線部を以下の語句に置き換えなさい。

<u>返金を受けとる</u>のにどのくらいかかるでしょうか。
〈私の歯をクリーニングする〉
<u>私の歯をクリーニングする</u>のにどのくらいかかるでしょうか。

1. 治療を終える
2. 私の治療を終える
3. そのクラウンの治療が終る
4. 予約を取る
5. 歯を形成する
6. 磨き方を覚える
7. 予約を取りなおす
8. プラークを除去する
9. そのアマルガム充填を終える
10. クラウンを作る
11. 私の歯を修復する
12. 保険会社からお金を受け取る

V. Substitute the following expressions in the example sentence.

Even <u>foreigners</u> are troubled by <u>the high value the yen</u>.
⟨cats/pollution⟩
Even <u>cats</u> are troubled by <u>pollution</u>.

1. horses/periodontal disease
2. royalty/dental disease
3. toothbrush manufacturers/tooth decay
4. dogs/tooth decay
5. dentists/toothaches
6. rich people/periodontal disease
7. farmers/pollution
8. Japanese/crime
9. children/bad breath
10. my cat/dental diseases
11. sugar bugs/toothbrushes
12. the police/tooth decay

Ⅴ．例文の下線部を以下の語句に置き換えなさい。

外国人だって円高で困っています。
〈猫／公害〉
猫だって公害で困っています。

1. 馬／歯周病
2. 王族／歯の病気
3. 歯ブラシ製造業者／むし歯
4. 犬／むし歯
5. 歯医者／歯痛
6. お金持ち／歯周病
7. 農家の人々／公害
8. 日本人／犯罪
9. 子どもたち／口臭
10. 私の猫／歯の病気
11. 砂糖の虫／歯ブラシ
12. 警官／むし歯

Chapter 9

Billing

Could You Send the Bill to My Office?

Although it is best to have the patient pay at the time the treatment is done, he may sometimes have you bill his office. Arrangements for billing should be done before the treatment begins. Make sure that you have the address for sending the statement.

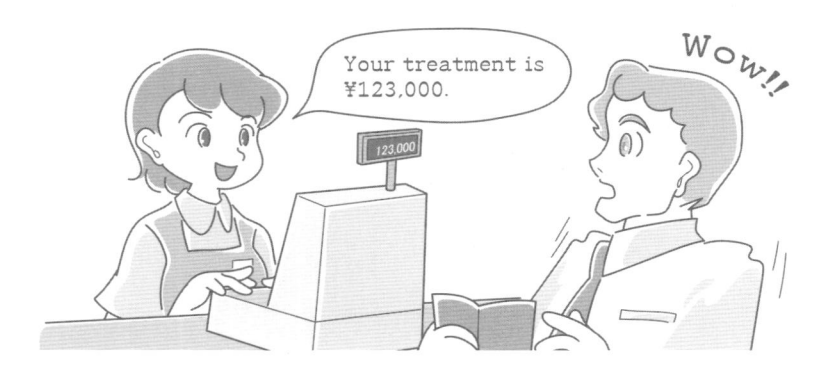

第 9 章

請求業務

請求書は私の事務所の方に送っていただけますか？

　患者には、治療が終った時点で支払ってもらうのが一番よいが、事務所の方に請求するように頼まれることもあるかもしれない。請求に関する取り決めは、治療を始める前にするべきである。また、必ず計算書を送る住所を知っておかなければならない。

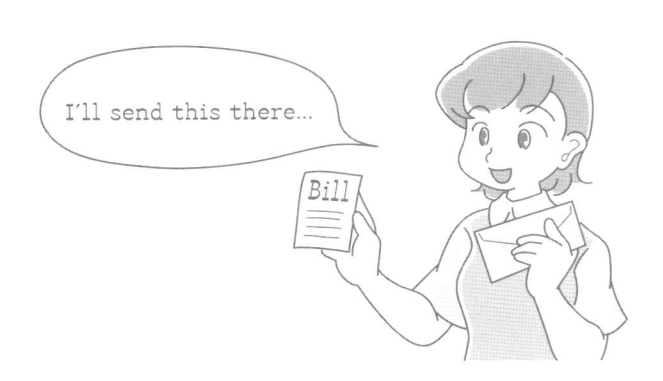

Situation: Ms. Fouget, an employee of the European Common Market office in Tokyo, is discussing having the bill for treatment sent to her.

Ms. Ishii: The doctor's estimate for your treatment is ¥123,000. This includes the examination, cleaning, three fillings, and one crown.
Ms. Fouget: That's a lot of money. Could you send a bill to my office?
Ms. Ishii: Certainly. Dr. Tanaka has already told me to send the bill there.
Ms. Fouget: Most dentists want to be paid in cash.

Ms. Ishii: That is true. We usually do that here. However, we have had several patients from your office and there has never been any trouble with payment.

Ms. Fouget: It certainly saves me a lot of trouble.
Ms. Ishii: Yes. It is a lot of money with the exchange rate being so high these days.
Ms. Fouget: You have my office address, don't you?
Ms. Ishii: Yes. We have it right here in the chart.

場面：東京のEC事務所に勤めるフォージェさんは、治療の請求書を送ってもらうことについて話しあっている。

石井さん：先生の治療の見積りは12万3千円です。これには、診査、クリーニング、充填が3つとクラウンが1つ含まれています。

フォージェさん：大きな金額ですね。請求書は私の事務所の方に送っていただけますか。

石井さん：かしこまりました。田中先生から、そちらに請求書を送るように言われております。

フォージェさん：ほとんどの歯医者さんはキャッシュで支払いをしてほしいようですが。

石井さん：そのとおりです。ここでも普通はそうしています。でも、フォージェさんの事務所からの患者さんが何人かいらっしゃいますが、今までお支払いに関して何も問題がありませんでした。

フォージェさん：それでずいぶん助かりますわ。

石井さん：ええ。最近の為替レートは高いので大きな金額になりますね。

フォージェさん：私の事務所の住所はおわかりですね。

石井さん：はい。このカルテに入っております。

Exercises

I. Substitute the following expressions in the example sentence.

Make sure that you <u>have the address</u>.
⟨call for an appointment⟩
Make sure that you <u>call for an appointment</u>.

1. confirm the appointment
2. talk with the receptionist
3. read the treatment plan
4. understand the treatment
5. talk with the dentist
6. bring your health insurance card
7. bring the X-rays with you
8. arrive on time
9. understand the billing procedures
10. send the recall card
11. brush
12. know how to floss

II. Substitute the following expressions in the example dialogue.

- The doctor's estimate for your treatment is <u>¥123,000</u>.
- That's a lot of money.
⟨¥70,000 (seventy thousand yen)⟩
- The doctor's estimate for your treatment is <u>¥70,000</u>.

練習問題

Ⅰ．例文の下線部を以下の語句に置き換えなさい。

必ず住所を知っていなければならない。
〈予約のために電話する〉
必ず予約のために電話しなければならない。

1. アポイントを確かめる
2. 受付係と話す
3. 治療計画を読む
4. 治療を理解する
5. 歯科医と話す
6. あなたの健康保険証を持ってくる
7. エックス線写真を持ってくる
8. 時間どおりに着く
9. 請求業務のやり方を理解する
10. リコールカードを送る
11. ブラッシングする
12. フロッシング方法を知っている

Ⅱ．例にあげた対話の下線部を以下の語句に置き換えなさい。

－先生の治療の見積りは12万3千円です。
－大きな金額ですね。
〈7万円〉
－先生の治療の見積りは7万円です。

− That's a lot of money

1. ¥86,000 (eighty-six thousand yen)
2. ¥53,000 (fifty-three thousand yen)
3. ¥1,000,000 (one million yen)
4. ¥524,000 (five hundred twenty-four thousand yen)
5. ¥125,000 (one hundred twenty-five thousand yen)
6. ¥62,500 (sixty-two thousand five hundred yen)
7. ¥87,000 (eighty-seven thousand yen)
8. ¥55,000 (fifty-five thousand yen)
9. ¥155,000 (one hundred fifty-five thousand yen)
10. ¥19,000 (nineteen thousand yen)
11. ¥28,000 (twenty-eight thousand yen)
12. ¥73,000 (seventy-three thousand yen)

Ⅲ. Substitute the following expressions in the example sentence.

The doctor will give you an estimate for the treatment.
〈treatment plan〉
The doctor will give you an estimate for the treatment plan.

1. crown
2. bridge
3. cleaning appointments
4. total treatment
5. implant
6. dentures

−大きな金額ですね。

1. 8万6千円
2. 5万3千円
3. 100万円
4. 52万4千円
5. 12万5千円
6. 6万2千5百円
7. 8万7千円
8. 5万5千円
9. 15万5千円
10. 1万9千円
11. 2万8千円
12. 7万3千円

Ⅲ．例文の下線部を以下の語句に置き換えなさい。

先生が治療の見積りを渡すでしょう。
〈治療計画〉
先生が治療計画の見積りを渡すでしょう。

1. クラウン
2. ブリッジ
3. クリーニング・アポイント
4. 治療全体
5. インプラント
6. 義歯

7. periodontal surgery
8. partial denture
9. extractions
10. fillings
11. restorations
12. emergency treatment

IV. Substitute the following expressions in the example sentence.

You have my <u>office address</u>, don't you?
⟨phone number⟩
You have my <u>phone number</u>, don't you?

1. home address
2. office phone number
3. records
4. X-rays
5. child's records
6. health history
7. new address
8. bill
9. treatment plan
10. husband's records
11. card
12. new phone number

7. 歯周外科
8. 部分義歯
9. 抜歯
10. 充填
11. 修復
12. 緊急治療

Ⅳ．例文の下線部を以下の語句に置き換えなさい。

私の<u>事務所の住所</u>はおわかり（お持ち）ですね。
〈電話番号〉
私の<u>電話番号</u>はおわかり（お持ち）ですね。

1. 自宅の住所
2. 事務所の電話番号
3. 記録
4. エックス線写真
5. 子どもの記録
6. 既往歴
7. 新しい住所
8. 請求書
9. 治療計画
10. 夫の記録
11. 名刺
12. 新しい電話番号

V. Substitute the following expressions in the example dialogue.

− Could you send a bill to my <u>office</u>?
− Certainly.
⟨home address⟩
− Could you send a bill to my <u>home address</u>?
− Certainly.

1. home
2. husband
3. office address
4. company
5. employer
6. address in America
7. wife
8. new address
9. old employer
10. father
11. father's office
12. bank

Ⅴ．例にあげた対話の下線部を以下の語句に置き換えなさい。

－請求書は私の事務所の方に送っていただけますか。
－かしこまりました。
〈自宅の住所〉
－請求書は私の自宅の住所の方に送っていただけますか。
－かしこまりました。

1. 自宅
2. 夫
3. 事務所の住所
4. 会社
5. 雇主
6. アメリカの住所
7. 妻
8. 新しい住所
9. 前の雇主
10. 父
11. 父の事務所
12. 銀行

Chapter 10

Transferring treatment records to the patient

Could I Have a Copy of My Dental Records?

Many of the foreigners in Japan stay here only a short time. They will ultimately return to their home countries and continue their dental treatment there. They will often ask for copies of their X-rays and records, together with recommendations for future treatment to be used by their dentist back home. Be sure to consult with the dentist before giving any X-rays or records to the patient.

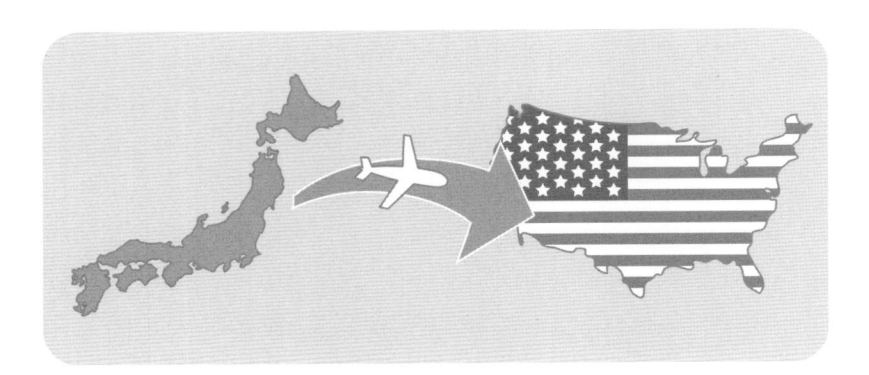

第 10 章

治療記録を患者に渡す

私の歯科記録のコピーをいただけますか？

　日本に住む外国人は、短い間だけの滞在であることが多い。最終的には本国に帰り、そこで歯科治療を続けることになる。彼らは、本国の歯科医が将来の治療のために使えるように、エックス線写真や記録のコピーを、今後の治療の勧めと共に求めることが多い。エックス線写真や記録を患者に渡す前に、必ず歯科医に相談しなければならない。

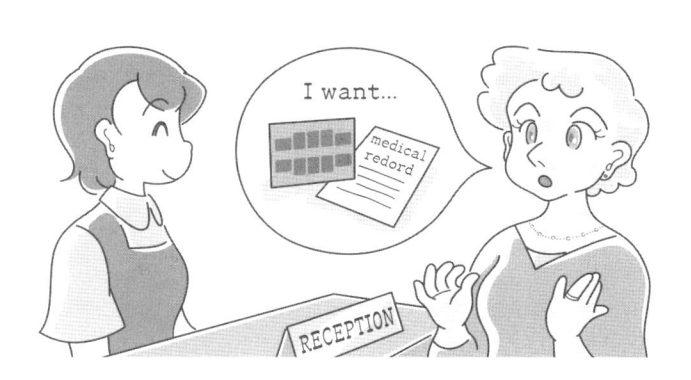

Situation: The Lewis family will be returning to the United States after living five years in Tokyo. The mother is asking about getting the X-rays and records.

Mrs. Lewis: We will be returning to the United States in one month and would like to get our dental records so we can continue treatment there.

Ms. Moriguchi: The doctor mentioned this to me. I am sorry to see you go.

Mrs. Lewis: We are sad to leave, but the children are getting older and it will probably be good for them to get into the American system of education.

Ms. Moriguchi: I will make a copy of your dental records and give you the X-rays.

Mrs. Lewis: That would be very nice.

Ms. Moriguchi: Also, it seems that your husband still needs some treatment.

Mrs. Lewis: Yes. He is always busy and never has time to take care of his teeth.

Ms. Moriguchi: Dr. Yamazaki will write a letter for the next dentist giving the treatment plan and the details of what needs to be done.

Mrs. Lewis: Thank you. That would be very kind. Also, could you give me the name of the dentist in Los Angeles who is Dr. Yamazaki's friend?

Ms. Moriguchi: Certainly. His name is Dr. Young. He is a fine dentist and teaches at the dental school there.

場面：ルイス家の人々は、東京に5年間いた後、アメリカに帰ることになっている。母親はエックス線写真と記録をもらうことについて尋ねている。

ルイス夫人：1ヵ月したらアメリカに帰ることになっていますので、そこで治療が続けられるように、私たちの歯科記録をいただきたいのですが。

森口さん：そのことは、先生からお聞きしております。お帰りになってしまうのは大変残念です。

ルイス夫人：私たちも、ここを出るのは悲しいのですけれど、子どもたちも大きくなってきますし、アメリカの学校に入る方が多分よいでしょう。

森口さん：歯科記録のコピーを作って、エックス線写真をお渡しします。

ルイス夫人：そうしてくださるとありがたいですわ。

森口さん：それから、ご主人様はまだいくらか治療が必要なようですね。

ルイス夫人：ええ。主人はいつも忙しくって、歯をケアする時間がないんです。

森口さん：山崎先生がご主人様の次の歯医者さんに、治療計画と必要なことの詳細を書いた手紙をお書きします。

ルイス夫人：ご親切にありがとうございます。それから、山崎先生のお友達のロサンゼルスの歯医者さんのお名前をいただけますかしら。

森口さん：かしこまりました。ヤング先生です。とても立派な歯科医で、そこの歯学部で教えていらっしゃいます。

Mrs. Lewis: I would appreciate that. We have never lived in Los Angeles. I dread trying to find a new dentist in a strange town.

ルイス夫人：ありがとうございます。私たちはロサンゼルスに住んだことがなくて、知らない町で新しい歯医者さんをみつけるのは不安なんです。

Exercises

Ⅰ. Substitute the following expressions in the example sentence.

Be sure to consult with the <u>dentist</u>.
⟨hygienist⟩
Be sure to consult with the <u>hygienist</u>.

1. nurse
2. receptionist
3. dental assistant
4. orthodontist
5. pedodontist
6. husband
7. father
8. mother
9. employer
10. secretary
11. laboratory technician
12. professor

Ⅱ. Substitute the following expressions in the example sentence.

We will be returning to <u>the United States</u> in one month.
⟨London⟩
We will be returning to <u>London</u> in one month.

練習問題

Ⅰ．例文の下線部を以下の語句に置き換えなさい。

必ず<u>歯科医</u>に相談しなければならない。
〈歯科衛生士〉
必ず<u>歯科衛生士</u>に相談しなければならない。

1. 看護師
2. 受付係
3. 歯科助手
4. 矯正歯科医
5. 小児歯科医
6. 夫
7. 父
8. 母
9. 雇主
10. 秘書
11. 技工士
12. 教授

Ⅱ．例文の下線部を以下の語句に置き換えなさい。

私たちは1ヵ月したら<u>アメリカ</u>に帰ることになっています。
〈ロンドン〉
私たちは1ヵ月したら<u>ロンドン</u>に帰ることになっています。

1. Belgium
2. Canada
3. Mexico
4. Norway
5. Germany
6. the head office
7. Spain
8. Argentina
9. Columbia
10. France
11. Paris
12. Rome

Ⅲ. Substitute the following expressions in the example sentence.

It seems that he still needs <u>some treatment</u>.
⟨a crown⟩
It seems that he still needs <u>a crown</u>.

1. a toothbrush
2. to brush his teeth
3. to have his teeth cleaned
4. to pay his bill
5. a filling
6. a dental examination
7. dental treatment
8. insurance

1. ベルギー
2. カナダ
3. メキシコ
4. ノルウェー
5. ドイツ
6. 本社
7. スペイン
8. アルゼンチン
9. コロンビア
10. フランス
11. パリ
12. ローマ

Ⅲ．例文の下線部を以下の語句に置き換えなさい。

彼はまだ<u>いくらか治療</u>が必要なようですね。
〈クラウン〉
彼はまだ<u>クラウン</u>が必要なようですね。

1. 歯ブラシ
2. 自分の歯を磨くこと
3. 歯をクリーニングしてもらうこと
4. 請求書の支払いをすること
5. 充填
6. 歯科診査
7. 歯科治療
8. 保険

9. more treatment
10. to see an orthodontist
11. to receive a letter of introduction
12. more fillings

Ⅳ. Substitute the following expressions in the example sentence.

He is always busy and never has time to take care of his <u>teeth</u>.
〈dental health〉
He is always busy and never has time to take care of his <u>dental health</u>.

1. periodontal problem
2. TMJ problem
3. children's teeth
4. oral hygiene problem
5. sore gums
6. painful tooth
7. toothache
8. dental appointments
9. dental records
10. dental X-rays
11. denture problems
12. dental needs

9. 治療がもっと
10. 矯正歯科医に診てもらう
11. 紹介状を受け取ること
12. 充填がもっと

Ⅳ．例文の下線部を以下の語句に置き換えなさい。

彼はいつも忙しくって、歯をケアする時間がないんです。
〈歯の健康〉
彼はいつも忙しくって、歯の健康をケアする時間がないんです。

 1. 歯周病の問題
 2. TMJの問題
 3. 子どもたちの歯
 4. 口腔衛生の問題
 5. 歯ぐきの痛み
 6. 痛い歯
 7. 歯痛
 8. 歯科の予約（に気をつける）
 9. 歯科記録（に気をつける）
10. 歯科のエックス線写真
11. 義歯の問題
12. 歯科のニーズ

V. Substitute the following expressions in the example sentence.

I dread trying to find a new dentist.
⟨an apartment⟩
I dread trying to find an apartment.

1. another dentist
2. the dental records
3. the dental X-rays
4. an orthodontist
5. a periodontist
6. misplaced charts
7. copies of old dental records
8. a dentist in a strange town
9. pedodontist
10. a doctor
11. a new hygienist
12. an oral surgeon

Ⅴ．例文の下線部を以下の語句に置き換えなさい。

新しい歯医者をみつけるのは不安です。
〈アパート〉
アパートをみつけるのは不安です。

1. 他の歯科医
2. 歯科記録
3. 歯科のエックス線写真
4. 矯正医
5. 歯周病専門医
6. 置き忘れたカルテ
7. 古い歯科記録のコピー
8. 知らない町の歯科医
9. 小児歯科医
10. 医者
11. 新しい歯科衛生士
12. 口腔外科医

付録

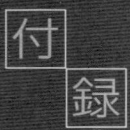

患者とのコミュニケーションで役立つ最重要用語100語

以下は、受付係と患者とのコミュニケーションに役立つ最重要用語100語を、アルファベット順に並べたものである。これらは歯科専門用語を知らない人にもわかる言葉である。

A

abscess	膿瘍
ache	痛む、痛み
address	住所
adjust	合わせる、調整する
amalgam	アマルガム
anesthetic	麻酔薬
antibiotics	抗生物質
appointment	予約、アポイント、約束
assistant	（歯科）助手

B

bill	請求書
braces	矯正装置
bridge	加工義歯

C

calculus	歯石
cancel	取り消す
cancellation	取り消し
cash	現金
cavity	むし歯、窩洞
charge	支払請求
chart	カルテ
checkup	（歯科）検診
cheek	頬
chief complaint	主訴
clean	（歯を）清掃する
cleaning	（歯の）清掃
clinic	診療所
condition	条件、状態
consultation	診察、相談
cost	費用

crown	歯冠、クラウン

D

decay	むし歯
dental	歯科の、歯の
dentist	歯科医
dentistry	歯科医学
denture	義歯

E

emergency	緊急
estimate	見積り
examination	予診、診査
examine	診察する
extract	抜く

F

fee	報酬、料金
fever	熱
filling	充填（物）
floss	フロス、糸
flossing	フロッシング

G

gums	歯ぐき

H

headache	頭痛
hygienist	衛生士

I

impression	印象
inflamed	炎症性の
inflammation	炎症
inlay	インレー
instructions	指示、指導
insurance	保険
introduction	紹介

L

laboratory	技工室、技工所
lower teeth	下顎の歯

M

molar	臼歯

O

office	診療所
operation	手術、処置
orthodontics	歯科矯正学
orthodontist	矯正歯科医

P

pain	痛み
pain killer	鎮痛剤
partial denture	局部義歯
patient	患者
pay	支払う
payment	支払い
pedodontist	小児歯科医

periodontal	歯周の
permanent tooth	永久歯
plaque	プラーク
porcelain	ポーセレン、陶材
prescription	処方箋
prevent	予防する
primary teeth	乳歯

R

recall	呼び戻す、リコール
receptionist	受付係
records	記録
reimburse	払い戻す、弁済する
restoration	修復、修復物
root canal treatment	根管治療

S

schedule	予定表
sensitivity	敏感
serious	重大な
specialist	専門医
surgery	外科学、外科
swelling	腫脹
swollen	腫れあがった

T

telephone number	電話番号
temporary	暫間の
toothache	歯痛
treat	治療する、処置する
treatment	治療、処置
treatment plan	治療計画
trouble	悩み、問題

U

upper tooth	上顎の歯
urgent	緊急の

W

waiting room	待合室
wisdom tooth	智歯

X

X-ray	エックス線

メモ

メモ

改訂版　クインテッセンス歯科英会話シリーズ
PART3 英語で話す歯科受付！

1989年10月30日　第1版第1刷発行
2007年10月10日　第2版第1刷発行

著　　者　　Thomas R. Ward
　　　　　　（トーマス　アール　ウォード）

発 行 人　　佐々木一高

発 行 所　　クインテッセンス出版株式会社
　　　　　　東京都文京区本郷3丁目2番6号　〒113-0033
　　　　　　クイントハウスビル　電話（03）5842-2270（代表）
　　　　　　　　　　　　　　　　　　（03）5842-2272（営業部）
　　　　　　　　　　　　　　　　　　（03）5842-2278（編集部）
　　　　　　web page address　http://www.quint-j.co.jp/

印刷・製本　サン美術印刷株式会社

©2007　クインテッセンス出版株式会社　　　　禁無断転載・複写
Printed in Japan　　　　　　　　　　　　落丁本・乱丁本はお取り替えします
　　　　　　　　　　　　　　　　　　ISBN978-4-87417-976-5　C3047
定価はカバーに表示してあります